Praise for *A Nurse's Story*

"In a post-SARS world where nurses are finally being recognized for the heroes they always were, *A Nurse's Story* is the best-seller no one can put down." — Montreal *Gazette*

"There are genuinely heart-rending, disturbing and thought-provoking stories to be found in the pages of *A Nurse's Story*. If this book doesn't give you pause, you're made of stone." — *Edmonton Journal*

"Tilda Shalof's *A Nurse's Story* is the first time the work of nurses has been documented in print in Canada in such an honest, no-holds-barred account. . . . Shalof has seen it all, and writes about it, too." — *Calgary Herald*

"[Shalof's] book isn't a doom-and-gloom account of overworked nurses. Interspersed with tales of tragedy are accounts of the funny, often bizarre events that transpire in an ICU." — *Canadian Press*

"[*A Nurse's Story* is] difficult to put down, so compelling and beautifully written are these stories. . . . Shalof's colleagues point out during one of their ongoing discussions about the value of their work, that eventually everyone needs a nurse. And for that reason alone, *A Nurse's Story* would be worth reading, in order to understand where it is most of us will end up sooner or later, what it is that might be visited upon us and just who it is that will be looking after us." — *Winnipeg Free Press*

"Readers may approach this book with the hope of reading dramatic tales such as those seen on television shows such as *ER*. While such readers are not likely to be disappointed, they are likely to discover more than they had hoped." — *Brandon This Week*

"A cracking good read. . . . I hope it's not the only story Shalof has to tell." — *Quill & Quire*

THE MAKING OF A NURSE

THE MAKING
OF A NURSE

TILDA SHALOF

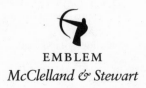

EMBLEM
McClelland & Stewart

Hardcover edition published 2007
Emblem edition published 2008

Emblem is an imprint of McClelland & Stewart Ltd.
Emblem and colophon are registered trademarks of McClelland & Stewart Ltd.

Library and Archives Canada Cataloguing in Publication

Shalof, Tilda
The making of a nurse / Tilda Shalof.

ISBN 978-0-7710-8095-1 (bound).– ISBN 978-0-7710-7983-2 (pbk.)

1. Shalof, Tilda.   2. Nurses – Canada – Biography.   3. Nursing –
Anecdotes.   I. Title.

RT37.S53A3 2007   610.73'092   C2006-904283-7

We acknowledge the financial support of the Government of Canada
through the Book Publishing Industry Development Program and that
of the Government of Ontario through the Ontario Media Development
Corporation's Ontario Book Initiative. We further acknowledge the
support of the Canada Council for the Arts and the Ontario Arts Council
for our publishing program.

Typeset in Sabon by M&S, Toronto
Printed and bound in Canada

This book is printed on acid-free paper that is 100% recycled,
ancient-forest friendly (100% post-consumer recycled).

McClelland & Stewart Ltd.
75 Sherbourne Street
Toronto, Ontario
M5A 2P9
www.mcclelland.com

4   5   12   11   10   09

CONTENTS

PREFACE

There are many wonderful things about writing a book, but the best, by far, is having readers and being in contact with many of them. Since the publication in 2004 of *A Nurse's Story*, I have heard from people all over the world. Many are nurses themselves who, despite a diversity of experiences and cultures, and the wide variety of roles, settings, and specialties in which they work, tell me that my nursing stories resonate strongly with theirs. In turn, these new conversations and connections have furthered my thinking about the journey of becoming a nurse and what it means to be a caregiver. Thus, *The Making of a Nurse* is both the story behind *A Nurse's Story*, as well as an up-to-the-minute follow-up of what nursing is like for me, still in it after twenty-five years. It is also my response to the many readers who have asked me to explain what I meant when I said I had to learn "to conquer myself in order to be of service to others." It was a phrase I had heard in a eulogy delivered at the funeral of a woman who had been a grandmother, a wife, a friend to many, and an active volunteer in the community. That phrase caught my attention because it seemed to sum up what I had been trying to accomplish both in my personal life and in my professional career.

During my childhood, both of my parents had serious, chronic illnesses. For years, I was their nurse, but as a teenager, I began to grow resentful of the care-giving responsibilities expected of me. I longed to escape what felt like an onerous burden. Then, of all things, I decided to study nursing. I remember the day I received my degree and my licence to practise and thought that was that: I was a nurse. *Hardly.* I had to be *made* into one. The patients I have cared for and the nurses I have worked with helped me become the nurse I aspired to be. (There are times when it still feels like a work in progress.)

While most practising nurses have expressed a familiarity with my stories, and indeed express a sense of affirmation to see many of them for the first time in print, other readers tell me that they have provided a window into a world they had never known about nor had the opportunity to enter. There is indeed a motherlode of nursing stories, however, and few have been recorded. I wanted to tell mine, but I had to find a way to do so that would ensure the utmost protection of patient privacy and confidentiality. So, once again, in *The Making of a Nurse*, I changed names (with the exceptions of my family, Pearl Bernard, Dr. Margaret Herridge, and nurse Janet Hale) and all unique and identifying details, and in a few cases created character composites, in order to ensure the complete anonymity of all patients and colleagues. My objective is to explore themes and issues that are not exclusive or particular to any individual patient, situation, or person, rather than to document specific character portraits.

To be honest, something else motivated me to write this book. I am worried. Some of the best nurses I know have left the profession, disillusioned and disheartened (there are lots of things that can wear you down!), and so many nurses actively discourage their own children from choosing nursing. At the same time, people in hospitals and in their own homes are in desperate need of more nursing care. There is a growing, worldwide shortage of nurses. If this trend continues, it will have an impact on each and every one of us: we will all need a nurse at some point in our lives. We are going to have to take very good care of ourselves so that we can take care of each other. Perhaps knowing what nursing is really like, at least from one nurse's perspective, will help people make a more informed choice about the profession. I hope this book contributes to that understanding.

I often wonder: Who would want to be a nurse, especially if they knew what it really entails? Who chooses nursing these days and why? I ask these questions honestly and open-mindedly, not rhetorically or cynically. Nursing is not a career you can advise or persuade someone to choose and it is a hard path to champion if you have not personally experienced its many satisfactions. I'm quite sure that the vast majority choose it because of a genuine desire to help others, but one nursing student told me nursing attracted him because "the salary is decent and it's steady work." Another told me she really wanted medicine, but didn't get in and nursing was her fallback. I'm afraid these motivations aren't going to cut it when those nurses enter a patient's room and are faced with raw human suffering. Nursing is dirty, gritty, messy, grinding, brutal, rough, and heartbreaking. It is also inspiring, sophisticated, challenging, fun, comforting, and at times, exhilarating.

I recall one day, years ago, sitting at the back of a hot, stuffy classroom, learning theories and abstract concepts about nursing, and the professor saying blithely, "Nursing is about Life," and then pausing to add, "and Life is about Nursing." *How trite, how inane*, I thought, jotting down that line in my notebook anyway, just in case I might be tested on it. I was only half paying attention, mostly daydreaming, wondering if I had what it took to be a nurse. Recalling that comment today, I think, *how true, how insightful*. Yet, how hard won that understanding has been.

My friend Joy says every reader will find something to cry about in this book. It is my sincere hope that every reader will also find lots to laugh about, as well. After all, if Life and Nursing have taught me anything, it is that the two go hand in hand.

Tilda Shalof
March 2007

1

HOME REMEDIES

My patient's name is Joe, or so he says, and I am his nurse. His chart states his name as Zbigniew Zwiezynskow and under place of residence, there is merely a sad trio of letters: NFA – "no fixed address." He's in his mid-forties, admitted last night to the Intensive Care Unit, the ICU, with pneumonia. He's feverish, delirious, and so violent that he may try to kill me if I decide to release him from the restraints we've placed on his arms and legs. But medically, his condition is improving – no small thing here in the ICU, where all of the patients have life-threatening, catastrophic illnesses. We're full; each of our twenty-two beds is occupied. Attached to every patient are monitors, machines, and equipment and in every room there are sickening odours and horrific sights, but I hardly notice these things any more. I have learned how to go beyond it all, to see through it, push it gently aside and go straight to the person lying there in the bed.

Today, all day, Joe is my patient. His heartbeats, urine output, breaths, cough, skin, dirty fingernails, and wild, greasy hair are all my concern. I will enter his world and for the next twelve hours, minute by minute, I will dwell with him there.

It's taken me such a long time to get here.

The sheer math astounds me. Since becoming a nurse in 1983, I have put in thousands of twelve-hour shifts at many different hospitals. I have worked with thousands of nurses and hundreds of doctors and other professionals. I have taken care of tens of thousands of patients ranging in age from eight to 104 who have had a multitude of diseases, illnesses, and injuries, and have administered to them a sea of intravenous fluids, rivers of syrups, suspensions, injectable medications, and at least a million pills, capsules, and tablets. Researchers study large populations, searching for patterns and trends, but the only way I know how to practise as a nurse is one patient at a time, seeing each individual in my care through illness, loss, pain, grief, or the prospect of death. For me, each time, the numbers all come down to one. As a nurse, there is the patient I am caring for and together, we proceed, one on one, side by side.

It wasn't always like this. Even though I was practically born a nurse, with strong instincts to help others, I was raw and unskilled; I had to be *made* into one. But long before it became my livelihood, taking care of others was my way of life. You could say I practised as an amateur for many years before going professional. My mother was my first patient and I cannot recall a time when I did not know it was my job to be her nurse. I was six years old when she first became ill, but as my father always said, I was very mature for my age.

WHENEVER SHE STARTED SHRIEKING, I went running. With her arms outstretched and her head flung back, crashing waves of sound poured out of her wide-open mouth. Her voice engulfed me. I was drowning, but I dove in to save her. "Please stop!" I screamed at her.

"I sing for you," she warbled.

"Don't!" I closed her lips with my fingers, but they exploded open again. Her voice filled the house. There was nowhere to hide. Low and rumbling one minute, it would suddenly screech up to a piercing high note. As soon as I was trapped by her voice, she would pause to recount one of her fables.

"When I was your age, I sang to the birds in the trees and they sang back to me." She returned to *Vissi d'arte*, then paused again. "I don't merely sing Tosca, I *am* Tosca." She gave a little laugh. "I am so Tosca, it's not funny. Like her, I live, and am prepared to die – for my art."

Yes, she was so Tosca, it made my head ache!

"Tosca brings me to the brink of madness." Her eyes shone. "Just to the brink, mind you."

Oh no, never further than that!

"And the secret to life, Tilda," she leaned forward to impart her wisdom, "is perfect breath control and deep diaphragmatic breathing."

Her life lessons were often interrupted by my three older brothers, especially when they trooped in together, always hungry, after school. "What's for dinner?" they'd ask. Tall high-school basketball star David was from my father's first marriage. Aloof, ambitious Stephen and angry, brooding Robbie were from my mother's first marriage.

"*Vichyssoise* and *bouillabaisse*," she sang, to the tune of *L'elisir d'amore*. On other nights it might be Chicken Cacciatore to *Le nozze di Figaro* or Bratwurst and Sauerkraut to *Der Rosenkavalier*. Her singing voice was like a signal to my brothers to vamoose. They scattered in different directions to their rooms, but I stayed close by her side.

She sang wherever and whenever the impulse struck her, even in the grocery store or at the bank. Big, cartoon blasts of Italian arias, French chansons, German Lieder ballooned out of her mouth. I flushed with shame. It was so annoying, so *unnecessary*. What would make her stop? Poison? A bullet? A dagger? I could do nothing but wait it out. She sang until she dropped down onto the couch in exhaustion. What a relief that was – like when the dentist stopped drilling. I wished she would stop altogether. Singing, I mean. She sang for friends at salon evenings in our home hosted by my father. It was at one such gathering that they each made an important announcement.

After her final encore, their friends called out, "Bravo, bravo!"

"Brava, brava," my father shouted, loudest of all, to correct them. He stood beside my mother at the piano and faced the guests. "What a set of pipes on that gal!" he crowed. "Unfortunately, Elinor hasn't been her best lately. The top medicos in the city are running a battery of tests, but I say all she needs is rest. She's wearing herself out taking care of the kids. They're a handful, especially Robbie. He's been acting up lately, nothing serious mind you, just normal teenage hijinks. David, what an athlete, and Stephen, what an outstanding scholar, and of course, Tilda is our little nurse. She's an angel. I don't know how we would manage without her." He put one arm around me and the other around my mother. "But Dr. Wilhemina DeGroot, the brilliant and renowned Chief of Neurology at Toronto General Hospital, is working on this most perplexing case. I feel certain she will come up with a magic pill."

My mother tugged on my father's sleeve, to indicate she wanted to say something. First, she thanked the guests, as she always did, but that night added something new. "This will be my last performance. If it were not for you, dear friends, I would not have the courage to go on."

"Of course you would, Ellie," my father interrupted. "You can beat this thing." The guests' voices rose up again and the tinkling of wineglasses merged with their conversation and laughter.

The next morning, I sat at the kitchen table with my brothers, each one barricaded behind their own cereal box, eating breakfast and planning for prizes they were going to send off for. My father had already left early to go to work. My mother appeared at the door, wanting to join us, but frozen in place. Her dark, wavy hair was tousled from sleep and she still had on her bright red lipstick and dark eyeliner from last night's performance and her black silk "Madama Butterfly" robe with pink blossoms swirling all over it. I jumped up and went to her. She leaned on me to make her way to the table, and when we got there, I eased her down onto a chair.

"Today," she announced, "I feel normal." No one was listening. "Well, *nearly* normal." From the pocket of her kimono she took out a small tin of blackcurrant lozenges and popped one into her mouth. She kept those purple "pastilles" close at hand to keep her lubricated so she could break into song whenever necessary. She cleared her throat. "I may have to cancel performances. I must shepherd my vocal resources." She glanced at the clock on the stove. "Aren't you kids late for school?"

Why didn't she know it was summer vacation?

Suddenly, she turned around in the chair as if someone was calling her. Was it a chorus of merry villagers? Don Giovanni asking for her hand in marriage? She stared at the chart on the stove and began to sing, "Beef, *boeuf*, 375 degrees; chicken, *poulet*, 375 degrees; ham, *jambon*, 375 degrees; veal, *veau*, 375 degrees; la, la la."

Robbie turned on the radio and strummed his index fingers in an agitated drumbeat to accompany the Rolling Stones, making it perfectly clear that Mick Jagger was not the only one around who could get no satisfaction. "What do you think of his voice?" he asked our mother.

His question broke her reverie. "Voice? You call that a voice? He has no voice. Singers nowadays can't make a sound without their moog synthesizers and microphones. They don't know the first thing about proper breathing. Who can understand a word he's wailing? His diphthongs are atrocious."

We could barely hear her. Her batteries were running low. "Why are you whispering?" I asked.

"I have to protect my vocal cords. I am not a piano or a violin. You can't press my keys or pluck my strings. My voice is my instrument and I have to keep it in good working order."

I knew all about her voice, how it required hydration, lubrication, and nutrients and how smoke, cool drafts, and spicy foods were to be avoided. She clutched onto the kitchen table to pull herself up and out of the chair. "Now if you children will excuse me, I must prepare for my concert."

"What concert?" Stephen asked with suspicion. We never knew what to believe.

"A benefit concert for the Institute for the Blind."

"How 'bout for the deaf?" Stephen muttered, making Robbie and David chuckle.

My mother slowly made her way to the living room, gripping each piece of furniture as she went, and I followed closely behind. At the piano there was a bouquet of red roses given to her by her friends, but they were wilted because no one had thought to put them in water. "I'll do some light numbers to cheer up those poor blind folk," she told me. "Nothing too serious." She rifled through stacks of sheet music. "Perhaps 'Smoke Gets in Your Eyes'? Or, what about 'On a Clear Day You Can See Forever'?" She loved her joke so much that she started laughing hysterically and within moments, tears streamed down her face. She could go from zero to flat-out howling laughter in seconds! I loved it when she laughed. When she finally caught her breath, she looked around at the room, as if seeing it in a new way. "It's a fairyland!" she exclaimed, suddenly seeing a world that was enchanted and hopeful. She wiped her eyes with the sash from her kimono. "Laugh and the world laughs with you, cry and you cry alone," she said, putting a damper on all the fun. "I'll do 'Ah, Sweet Mystery of Life' and Schubert, of course."

Right then and there, I wanted to tell her that I loved her, but couldn't make my mouth form the words and I said nothing. Then she said she was tired, so I helped her over to the couch to lie down for a rest.

MY PARENTS WERE BOTH widows with young children when they met. My mother had been married to a New York lawyer, and one snowy evening while driving home, his De Soto turned over into a ditch. He died a few days later in the hospital.

"Overnight, I became a widow with two young songs – I mean *sons*," she told me once and giggled helplessly at her slip of the tongue.

One year later, Harry Shalof, also a widower, but fifteen years older than she and with a son of his own, started coming backstage at the concerts she gave, such as a fundraiser for the synagogue or an evening of Christmas carols in the church. A few months later they married and settled down in a sleepy little town in rural Pennsylvania where they had me. My father worked in a dry

cleaning plant and my mother stayed at home, substituting lulla-
bies for arias.

But in the early sixties, as the Vietnam War escalated, my father
felt a growing horror and shame. He decided to pack up and seek
haven in reasonable, peaceful Canada. He also wanted to protect
his sons from being drafted into the army. He moved us all to
Toronto, where he continued to watch the conflict every night on
TV. "War has become the American way," he lamented. "I could not
stay." My father found a job as a dry cleaning salesman and drove
all around the city and outlying suburbs, his car loaded up with
pressing irons, jugs of chemicals, and plastic bags. In the evenings,
after work, he loved to cook rich, strange foods, take night courses
at the university for the "mature" student, and in his spare time was
writing a book about stain removal entitled *Out, Damn Spot!*

MY MOTHER'S ILLNESS crept over her slowly. For a long time I had
had an inkling something was wrong with her mind, but now something was definitely wrong with her body. Which was worse? By
the time I was eight years old, I knew for sure she was sick, both
inside and out. I wondered if she would die and how I would feel if
she did. I felt there might be some advantages to me if she did die,
but of course, I told myself, I didn't want her to. *Of course not.*

"Sometimes your mother needs a bit of help with her ADL,"
explained my father on days when he asked me to stay home from
school to help her. By then I knew the medical jargon for the
"Activities of Daily Living." ADL meant, for example, going to
the bathroom. To get her there, I walked backwards, facing her
while she held on to my forearms for balance and momentum.
I waited outside the door, listening for when she was done, and
then went in to get her. She also needed a boost getting up from
the couch or a prod to start moving from a standing position.
Sometimes she would even break into a run of a few tiny steps and
then stop abruptly, as if someone had yelled, "Freeze!" I was there
to catch her when she fell, which happened often. For no appar-
ent reason, she would stumble or trip over nothing at all and
crumple to the floor.

"I can't seem . . . to get my balance." She clutched the air as I pulled her up from the kitchen floor one time. "I'm having an off day."

Most of the time, she lay on the couch, spilling over the edges. When she stood up, it was strange to see her vertical. In every moment, with every movement, I was with her. I knew her feelings, her very thoughts. When she was sad, I was sad. When her spirits lifted, my heart soared. It felt cruel to be happy around her, as if I was mocking her, so I tried not to be too energetic or flaunt my robust health in front of her.

"There are days when I can hardly manage to create a sound and other days when I feel miraculously reborn," she told me.

Some days she seemed to cast off her illness. "Let's go window shopping," she might say, her voice suddenly audible. "How about a drive in the country? I feel on top of the world." She held her head high and let loose with a few blasts of song. "No one can even tell there's anything wrong with me!"

By the next day she'd be sunk into the couch. "I'm not on today," she'd say. "It's an off day."

She was a light switch!

"It's the well-documented 'on-off syndrome,'" my father said. He had begun subscribing to medical journals.

But there began to be more off days than on. Days when she couldn't get out of bed and I stood beside her doling out her blue and yellow pills, holding a glass of water to her lips as she took them one by one, with long sighs in between each swallow.

When she spoke, you could hardly hear her. When she sang, she made the plates and cutlery jump on the table. Her hands trembled when she dialled the telephone, yet her handshake was powerful. She toppled over at the slightest disturbance like when the toast popped up or when the carpet gave off a crackle of static electricity. And at night, I knelt beside her and talked to her to calm her nerves and checked to make sure she was breathing. She fell asleep easily, but in the morning she always said how tired she was. It was as if sleeping exhausted her and being awake made her sick.

Let me switch with you. I'll be the sick one and you can be the healthy one. I can handle it.

My two older brothers David and Stephen kept their distance, but Robbie demanded answers. "Why do you lie down so much?" He stood looming over her where she lay, mired in the couch.

"I am tired but when I sing, I feel as light as a bird."

"Why did you have to get sick?"

"Believe me," she said behind closed eyes, "it wasn't my intention."

"What's wrong with you?"

"Robbie, stop pestering your mother." My father intervened. "She needs to rest."

His eyes narrowed. "What do you mean by that? Why don't you ever tell that to Tilda?"

"Tilda is your mother's nurse. She takes care of her."

Robbie had many questions, but if my father asked him, "Where are you going after school?" or "Will you be home for dinner?" he would answer with a scowl. Robbie cut classes, shoplifted, and got sent to the principal's office for swearing or smoking cigarettes. Usually he told me to get lost, but sometimes he wanted me to be with him all day and all night. "Til, you're the best sister anyone could ever have. I need you to stay close because I'm worried about my mind." He sat on the edge of his bed with his head in his hands. "I am ill," he said grimly. "Quite ill. Do not underestimate the quiteness of that ill."

I placed my palm on his forehead as if to take his temperature. I had no idea how to help him other than to love him. My father was busy with my mother's illness and couldn't take on more worries. David and Stephen went away to university and as soon as Robbie finished high school, he ran away and no one knew where. He wrote to me from Chicago, San Francisco, and then London, England. A few years later, he landed up in Israel, which seemed like a strange place to find peace, but there he seemed to, for a time, until he moved on to other ports of call.

"DON'T GO TO SCHOOL," my mother said one day that fall. "Stay home with me. I need you." She stretched out her arms to me. "I feel better when you are here." I had been missing a lot of school,

but my teachers didn't seem to mind. I lay down beside my mother
on my parents' rumpled bed, and we watched TV and ate marsh-
mallows. In the afternoon, I got up and walked around aimlessly,
feeling homesick. The house was dark, messy, and had a sour,
musty smell. Stacks of old newspapers were piled up and there were
dusty books everywhere. I couldn't wait to grow up and leave home
like my brothers. I went into the bathroom and examined myself in
the mirror. Looking back at me was just a sad, ordinary girl.

"Brown hair, green eyes. Average height and weight," the
school nurse had recorded on my chart that I snuck a peek at.
"Well-nourished. Brushes her teeth correctly."

"Shy. Introverted," the school's guidance counsellor had
written in my file that I read upside down, from the other side of
his desk. "Quiet and helpful."

"What do I look like?" I went back to the bed and asked my
mother.

"*Du bist wie eine Blume*," she trilled, clasping her hands to her
heart.

But I didn't want to be a blossom, or a ray of sunshine, nor a
star from the heavens above. I did not want to be an angel or
a nurse. I wanted to be a normal girl with a normal mother.

I got back on the bed beside her and resumed my ongoing
project of plucking out tufts of chenille nap from their olive-
coloured bedspread while watching *Gilligan's Island*, *Bewitched*,
and my favourite, *Dr. Ben Casey*. He was a neurosurgeon, played
by the gorgeous heartthrob Vince Edwards. The opening always
gave me chills when a disembodied hand appeared on the screen
and wrote the following symbols while a solemn voiceover intoned
the words: "man ♂, woman ♀, birth *, death †, and infinity ∞."
I sat, my eyes riveted to the screen, fingering the bedspread threads
and pretending they were the dark chest hairs sticking out of the
collar of Dr. Casey's white shirt, always open by one or two
buttons. That open shirt showed his maverick spirit as he battled
brain tumours and aneurysms and rebelled against the conserva-
tive medical establishment that tried to rein him in. He didn't
suffer fools gladly and was gruff and demanding, but he was a
dreamboat and besides, he had to be cruel to be kind, didn't he?

He dared to perform complicated operations that no one else would touch, even risking his own life once when he accidentally contaminated himself with a patient's needle. Gentle Nurse Wills was always at his side to soften the blow and to wipe the sweat from his brow during long operations. She was there, too, after hours, to help him take his mind off things, at least until the episode when he fell in love with a patient who had been in a coma for thirteen years, but awoke looking more beautiful than ever, every hair in place and her make-up on!

As soon as my mother fell asleep, I went out and walked to Shopper's Drug Mart. Once, I had noticed there large plastic bottles of big pink capsules filled with white gelatine powder, guaranteed to strengthen brittle fingernails. I bought a bottle and returned home. In the bathroom I emptied each capsule into the sink. I wrote messages on tiny marijuana rolling-papers I found in one of my brothers' rooms and inserted each one into an empty capsule. "Time for your medicine," I said, handing her one along with a glass of the purple loganberry juice that she loved. "Just what the doctor ordered. Miracle pills." I opened one and read it to her. "Today Is the First Day of the Rest of Your Life." Others read, "You Can Do It!" or "Keep on Truckin'" or "Every Day, in Every Way, You Are Getting Better." She was so excited she wanted to open them all, but I told her not to overdo it; she'd had enough for one day.

A few hours later, my father came home and got busy making dinner. I sat at the kitchen table and lost myself in the crazy whirling wallpaper that depicted jars of pickles, mustards and relishes, ham hocks and lamb chops, sheaves of wheat, and fruits and vegetables from every vine, tree, and bush, bursting forth out of straw cornucopias. My father heaved pots and frying pans onto the stove and soon his head became enveloped in a cloud of steam that fogged his glasses. Pots splattered and spluttered onto the enamel surface, and as he tasted from each one, he told me about his day. "If the customer doesn't tell the dry cleaner about the stain, they can't treat it. Home remedies are merely first aid, but dry cleaning saves the patient. Guess, what's the most stubborn stain?"

"Ink?"

"It's mustard!" he exclaimed. "It takes a lot of know-how to dry clean fabrics, and that's where Regal Sales excels. We've got the best products on the market." He went to get my mother and brought her to the kitchen, and we propped her up at the table. "Come on, Ellie, sit up straight!" he coached. He set bowls of steaming rice and chop suey in front of us. "Kung Hei Fat Choy," he said to welcome the Chinese New Year. "First, let's check your progress today." He flipped through the notes I'd made about whether my mother had done her exercises, what her heart rate and blood pressure had been, and if she had cried. He was pleased with her day. "Now, let's eat."

There were very few rules in our family, but one of them was chopsticks.

"Here Ellie, let me get you started." He positioned them in her hand.

"I'm sorry I'm so slow." My mother tried to grip the chopsticks, but they slithered away.

"Hold the top one like a pencil. That's it! Move it up and down. You'll get it."

But I could see that she couldn't grasp a thing so I moved my chair closer to hers and made a napkin into a bib and tied it around her neck. The chopsticks slipped out of her fingers and clattered to the floor. "No, Tilda, she can't give up," I heard my father say as I bent down to pick them up. I decided to stay down there awhile. Crouched under the kitchen table, I began to dream up a plan. I decided that if I would be a devoted and gentle nurse, the kindest, most attentive nurse possible, in return my mother would get well. While I was at it, I would be the most loving, understanding sister so I could make Robbie happy, too. And if I could be a doting, obedient daughter, I could ensure nothing bad would happen to my father.

Unfortunately, in the years that followed, not one of us kept our side of the bargain.

2

WATERGATE DIAGNOSIS

By the time I was eleven years old, I had a new patient to worry about.

Something was wrong with my father. Every night, long after midnight, I heard bizarre sounds. I crept into my parents' bedroom and found my father sitting on the edge of the bed, rubbing his chest. He had a strained look and in his hand he held a row of white antacid tablets – lined up like the pennies and nickels he rolled and took to the bank. He pounded lightly on his chest. "*Greppps . . .* ," I heard him say.

"What's wrong, Dad?"

"Not a thing, my dear. It's nothing but mild heartburn. *Greckkk . . .*"

"It seems your father has become a musical instrument. A woodwind," my mother said. She was lying beside him, waving an imaginary baton in the air. "He's playing *Eine Kleine Nachtmusik.*"

"It doesn't sound good, Dad." I stood there, staring and worrying.

"It's nothing but garden-variety borborygmi. Intestinal rumblings caused by moving gas."

"What does the doctor say?"

"Well, as a matter of fact I'll take you with me to my appointment next week. It will be an educational experience for you. Maybe you'll be a doctor one day?"

But he had taught me about rhetorical questions; you didn't have to answer them.

AT THE DOCTOR'S OFFICE my father went to the men's room and returned with a plastic container filled to the brim. He handed it to the nurse, saying jovially, "*Urine* the money!" She took it from him carefully. Then, she placed suction cups on his chest, and I stood watching as a needle on a machine rose and fell, sketching twelve different views of his heart on strips of pink graph paper. Next, the nurse drew blood from his arm, and my father beamed at the healthy-looking sample his body had produced. He held the test tube of blood in his hands and marvelled at its warmth. We moved to the examining room, where the doctor took his blood pressure, first one arm and then the other, first standing up and then lying down, and placed his stethoscope on my father's hairy chest, closed his eyes, and listened.

"Hear a symphony in there, Doc?" my father asked.

The doctor asked him to please be quiet, *please*, so that he could *auscultate* properly. "Have you had chest pain, Mr. Shalof? Palpitations? Indigestion?"

"No problems whatsoever. I've never felt better. It's my wife –"

"Frankly, there are some worrisome findings here. Nothing conclusive, but I would like to do some tests. In the meantime, I am putting you on a strict diet. You are overweight and that is putting a strain on your heart. Also, you have diabetes." He paused to look over at me. "Your daughter will have to be alert for signs of a precipitous drop in your blood sugar and be prepared to take action."

Yikes. What did that entail?

"A diet?" echoed my father as if he was unfamiliar with the word. "The great philosopher Montaigne said diets prepare one for death, that they undermine one's enjoyment of life."

"Cut back on the calories. Reduce your salt intake. No sugar. Low-fat."

"What's left?" He looked quizzical.

"Mr. Shalof, you're now in your sixties. Have you considered retirement?"

"Please, Doc, I'm a long way off from that." My father reeled back in mock horror. "Say, about those tests, can I study for them? Ha, ha . . ."

"First of all, a chest X-ray and more blood work. A barium enema – I know it's not the most pleasant thing – and I'd like you to see a colleague of mine, a cardiologist."

"*Barium*? Isn't that what you do with the patients who don't make it?" The doctor busied himself with the chart, but my father pressed on. "Hey, Doc, what's Italian for 'enema'?"

The doctor looked up.

"An *innuendo*! Get it?" A faint smile flickered across the doctor's lips, which only encouraged my father. "Say, if you jumble up the letters in 'laxative,' you get 'exit lava'! Pretty good, eh?"

"You can book the tests with my nurse," the doctor said, his back already to us as he opened the door to leave.

After the doctor's appointment, my father suggested we take a stroll through Queen's Park. "What a great city!" he exclaimed, gazing around as if at all of Toronto at once. "In New York's Central Park, you could get mugged. In the Damrak in Amsterdam, you'd get high from the dope fumes. Tilda, take a deep breath of our city's fresh air." He helped himself to one. "Enjoy our clean, safe streets."

I was quiet, brooding over what the doctor had said.

"Are you worried about missing school, Tilda?"

I nodded. *That too.*

"Some experiences in life are more educational than school." He studied me intently for a moment. "You really are so grown up."

That had always been my claim to fame.

I often wondered where the mythical truant officer lurked, the one who prowled the streets on the lookout for children playing hooky. I prayed he would find me and send me back to school. The principal and teachers knew there were problems at home and never questioned my frequent absences. My friend Joy thought I was lucky to miss so much school.

My father jangled his keys in his pocket as we stood on the subway platform waiting for the northbound train to take us home. "See, Tilda, that was one doctor's *opinion*. We'll go to other doctors and get more opinions. We'll make our own inquiries, come to our own conclusions."

I was busy thinking about the twelve ways of looking at the heart. My father was loving, oh yes, and good-hearted, and kind, and bossy, and I was afraid he was going to die.

MY TELEVISION TRAINING with Dr. Ben Casey, the neurosurgeon, turned out to be good preparation for my starring role accompanying my parents to doctor's appointments, especially my mother, to hers with Dr. DeGroot, Chief of Neurology at Toronto General Hospital. I went along to help with buttons, zippers, belts and boots, chairs, stairs, escalators, and furniture. The doctor was tall and severe-looking. She had the same serious expression and wore similar, drab clothes at each visit: a brown tweed skirt, a plain white blouse buttoned to the neck, a white lab coat with a slender silver reflex hammer sticking out of a pocket, and sturdy black oxfords. Her manner was stern and brusque, just like Dr. Ben Casey's, and she didn't waste anyone's time, especially her own.

"I think Willie DeGroot prefers the company of women, if you know what I mean," Dad told my mother with a wink, after the first appointment.

My mother put her trust in her. "I'll do whatever she says. She's the one who will help me."

"You can't do better than Chief of Neurology at a world-class *horse pistol*. Dr. DeGroot is the head honcho! Now, I'm all for Women's Lib, but it does take some getting used to."

Sometimes I took my mother to her appointments by myself. We went through the same routine at each visit. First, I would hand over to Dr. DeGroot the clipboard with all the charts my father had set up for me to log my observations of my mother's condition. The doctor would glance at them while my mother smiled at her coyly, as if by ingratiating herself she would be rewarded with a better diagnosis. Then I was expected to stand back and let her struggle solo through the rest of the exam. I felt like a traitor, as if I were letting her down. I was used to covering for her but now, in front of the doctor, her infirmity was exposed. From time to time, I lurched forward to offer my arm, but Dr. DeGroot waved me away. At the doctor's request, my mother took ten steps forward, ten backward, tried to hop on one leg, swung her arms over her head, scissored them at her sides, clapped her hands, one, two, three, sat down in a chair and then attempted to get up out of the chair by herself. She performed these actions with weak and faltering motions as if moving against resistance, like she was pulling her limbs through water.

Once, Dr. DeGroot brought in medical students to observe this interesting case. "Now, I will demonstrate the Babinski reflex," Dr. DeGroot said. She used a key to gently scratch the soles of my mother's bare feet. "Can you feel that, Mrs. Shalof?"

"I'm not dead *yet*." She rolled her eyes and smiled at the students, who appreciated her joke.

Dr. DeGroot went on to check her reflexes, her handgrips, tongue muscles, eyebrow movements, and her ability to identify samples of peppermint, lemon, and vanilla. "Testing the twelve cranial nerves is an essential part of a complete neurological examination," the doctor explained.

I thought of offering them the useful mnemonic my father had taught me to help remember those cranial nerves: "On Old Olympus Tiny Tops, a Finn and German Viewed Some Hops," for olfactory, optic, oculomotor, trochlear, trigeminal, abducens, facial, acoustic, glossopharyngeal, vagus, spinal, and hypoglossal. (He told me a racy version, too: "Oh, Oh, Oh, to Touch and Feel a Girl's Vagina, Such Heaven!")

"Now, Mrs. Shalof, I want you to write something for us." She handed her a pen and paper.

"What shall I write? A sonnet? An epistle? My last will and testament?"

"Anything will do. Why don't you make a list of your daily activities?"

The way my mother picked up the pen and positioned herself on the chair I saw immediately that she had become Tatiana, composing the letter to Eugene Onegin in Tchaikovsky's opera. Dr. DeGroot took a look at the page and passed it to the students, who nodded. "Micrographia," she said gravely.

Bingo! A point scored in the diagnosis game!

Dr. DeGroot explained to the students the complex process of examining the mind. "First, establish the patient's level of consciousness. It is the most sensitive indicator of neurological status. Then, observe whether the patient is alert, drowsy, confused, stuporous, or comatose. In a true coma, if you lift the eyelid it will gradually cover the eye. In a hysterical coma, the eye rapidly closes."

My mother blinked a few times to demonstrate that she was experiencing neither type of coma.

"Now, we will perform the functional inquiry to examine cognitive function. In other words, speak to the patient." She turned to the subject at hand. "How are you today, Mrs. Shalof?"

"Ever so much the better for your asking, Dr. DeGroot."

"Mrs. Shalof, can you please tell us in which direction the sun sets?"

I saw how desperately she wanted to give the correct answer, but was either confused or simply didn't know. She looked at me helplessly. Behind the doctor's lab-coated back, I mouthed the answer, but she had looked away.

"I always tell my children, don't let the sun set on your anger. Resolve your differences before the day is done." She saw from the doctor's frown that that wasn't the desired response.

How could she not know that the sun sets in the west? She knew every word of La forza del destino *and could name every aria that Renata Scotto had sung at her La Scala debut.* Sometimes I wondered if she was playing a game. Perhaps the joke was on us?

"Please count backwards from one hundred by threes, Mrs. Shalof."

"Higher mathematics has never been my strong suit."

Dr. DeGroot went on to check "expressive functions" by asking her to use words in a sentence, first *apple* and *donkey*, and then *microscope* and *guillotine*. When she got to *chattel* and *amanuensis*, my mother's energy flagged and her voice began to fade. We could hardly hear her.

"Now, I will test the patient's abstract reasoning," the doctor explained. "Mrs. Shalof, what does 'people who live in glass houses shouldn't throw stones' mean?"

Despite her fatigue, she sat up tall and tried her best. "It is a parable about resolving conflicts peacefully. It is never necessary to resort to violence."

"What about 'a rolling stone gathers no moss'?"

"Oh, the Rolling Stones! I can't stand their moaning and caterwauling. They are ruining their vocal cords. Oh, let's see. It's about discipline. Stay true to your dreams and you will succeed." She looked up hopefully into Dr. DeGroot's stern gaze. "Perhaps this is all a dream and there's nothing wrong with me. Is that possible?"

"You most definitely have a degenerative neurological condition." Dr. DeGroot washed her hands at a little sink and ushered us to the door. On the way out, I glanced back to see what my mother had written.

To Do

1.

2

3.

4. Dream

5.

By Mrs. Elinor Shalof

THERE WAS ANOTHER occasion when my father asked me to go with
my mother to her appointment because he had a business meeting.
Again, Dr. DeGroot put my mother through her paces. Afterwards,
the doctor stood washing her hands and looked back at us in the
little mirror over the sink and said, "You may get dressed now, Mrs.
Shalof. I have arrived at a diagnosis. Please wait outside until I call
you back in."

My mother turned to me to dress her. For the examination she
had worn a paper gown that flapped open at the back and a pair of
floppy paper slippers. As I put her clothes on her and zipped and
buttoned everything, I pretended she was a doll and we were playing
dress-up. We went out to the waiting room, where there was a television on that no one was watching. The Watergate investigation
was underway and it was on all the time, for weeks now, non-stop.
"Let's stay here and watch this. It takes my mind off my own problems." She pulled at my sweater to bring me down to sit beside her.
"Those guys are in worse trouble than I am." We sat watching and
after a few minutes, Dr. DeGroot called us back in. I offered my hand
to help my mother out of the chair, but she wouldn't budge. I tried
to pull her up. Her body was a tug of war between us.

"Come on, Dr. DeGroot wants to see you again." I yanked on
her arm. "Come on! Get up!"

"You go. Come back afterward and tell me what she said."

"Where is your father today?" the doctor asked when I returned
to her office.

"He couldn't make it. He had a meeting."

"Well, you seem very grown up for your age. What are you,
about thirteen, fourteen?"

"Twelve."

"You have a very close relationship with your mother, I can see
that." She looked sad, which seemed her way of being kind. "Your
mother is a fascinating case. Sit down, Tilda." She pointed to a chair.
"She has a serious brain disorder that is uncommon in a woman in
her mid-forties. It is likely a sequela of an infective encephalopathic
process that manifests in Parkinson's disease. In addition, she
exhibits a number of concomitant components of motor neuron
disease and cognitive and psychiatric derangement."

It sounded bad, though not nearly as bleak as when Dr. Ben Casey closed the patient's chart and sadly walked away. "Is it contagious?" I asked. *It felt like it was.*

"Of course not, but her condition is unusual. I will be publishing an account of her case history in the *Annals of Neurology.* Your father can read it in the next issue. Now, she's not too far gone yet, but she will get much worse. There is no cure, but there are medications for the symptoms and promising new developments on the horizon. Now, go out there and tell your mother what I've just told you and if she has any questions, bring her back."

What could I make of that mumbo-jumbo? At least it wasn't like when Dr. Ben Casey dropped a bombshell of "subarachnoid hemorrhage" or "astrocytoma, malignant, inoperable" and from his hard-set expression and dark eyes, you knew it was game over.

I went back out to the waiting room. The television flickered and the investigation droned on. The sad, grim faces of the Watergate men loomed large on the screen, reflecting the miserable faces of the patients sitting around the room, also worried about their fates. My mother was staring at the screen, still sitting in the chair where I had left her, her elbows cradled in her hands, held close like someone might take them from her. I thought about turning around and running away, never to return. *What if I leave her here? She's too much for me. I can't handle this!* I went over to her. Her eyes stayed fixed on the TV set as I repeated the doctor's words, but with a more upbeat delivery. She turned away and it looked as if she was crying, but there were no sounds or tears. "Are you okay?"

She shook her head, part yes, part no. "Dr. DeGroot said that with certain conditions, patients are not able to produce tears. I must have one of those." She wiped her face of tears that weren't there. "But believe me, it doesn't mean they don't cry. You can cry without tears. I can vouch for that." I sat down with her to watch the defendants with their shamed faces getting grilled about their devious activities. We laughed at the earnest men, their implausible alibis, and their circuitous explanations for obvious wrongdoings.

"And I thought *I* had problems," my mother said, and we laughed even more.

We sat in the waiting room until the Commission broke for
lunch. I helped her up out of the chair, and she leaned into me.
"My nerves are shot," she said softly. We walked slow, tiny steps
to the subway station, my mother clinging to me every inch of the
way. As the train roared into the station, she held on even tighter.
Suddenly, she swayed forward and I reached out to pull her back
from the edge. "Don't worry, I won't jump. I can't even whip
myself up into enough of a frenzy to commit suicide." She sank
into the nearest seat on the train and pulled me down beside her.

"We'll be home soon," I told her. *Please wait until we get there
before falling apart!*

She cuddled my arm and stroked it like it was a kitten. As soon
as we got home she was seized by a bolt of energy. She pushed me
aside and marched ahead, still in her coat and boots. She went into
the den where there was a hi-fi stereo and a metal rack filled with
record albums. She flipped through them and grabbed Maria
Callas singing Norma and Leontyne Price's Aïda. She pulled each
album out and cracked it over her knee. The brittle seventy-eights
broke easily, but the flexible LPs required more force. She looked
odd, standing on one leg, the other bent up high, like a flamingo.

"Don't break your records!" I pulled the pieces from her hands.

"Life is nothing to me if I can't sing."

"But Dr. DeGroot didn't say you wouldn't be able to sing."

"What does that numbskull know about music?" She plunged
her face into her hands. "I can't bear to listen to great voices and
be reminded that I can no longer produce my best. What is more
pathetic than the artist who can no longer perform? I might as well
be dead. Will you find a way to kill me?"

I took her hand, like Dr. Ben Casey's Nurse Wills did with a
patient after surgery. It might be "curtains" for the patient, but
the nurse always stayed at the patient's side, even after the doctor
left the scene. I put my mother to bed, imagining myself as part of
a long tradition of noble caregivers who kept vigils at the bedsides
of the infirm. I was Jo March from *Little Women*, who waited all
night for Beth's fever to break, but by morning Beth was gone.

"I feel better when you're with me." She snuggled up close.

"Don't go to school. Stay here. I need you more than that silly old school."

"What do you mean? Not go back? Quit school?"

"Why not?"

"It's against the law for one thing. I have to go back. I'll never catch up. I'm missing everything!" The only other kid I knew of who didn't go to school was Pippi Longstocking. I turned the TV on to keep my mother company and went downstairs to wait for my father to come home.

SLEEP USUALLY CAME so easily to me, but that night I lay there stewing until long after Johnny Carson's lead-in theme song and monologue. When it was over, my father got up and signed off, just like his favourite broadcaster, Walter Cronkite: "And that's the way it is, February 19, 1972." My mother came into my room and I pretended to be asleep.

"You awake?" she whispered. She slipped off her shoes and sunk down onto my bed. The darkness seemed to give her even more licence to nestle in close and seek comfort in my arms. I hated how she used my body to make hers feel better, the way one huddles around a fire for warmth. "If only I could be a better mother to you," she murmured.

Aha! Now, we were getting somewhere! I sat up eagerly. "What would you do?"

"I would give you the sun, the moon, and the stars."

But my wishes were so much more modest than that!

"Tilda, what would I do without you? Promise you'll never leave me. That you'll always take care of me." I nodded. "Will you make sure that nothing bad ever happens to me?"

"Yes," I pledged. "Of course." I saw no reason why not.

"I am embarking on a difficult course. It may be the fight of my life, but I am prepared to give everything so that I may sing again. I will need your help." She brought her lips to my ear. "And another thing," she whispered. "When the time comes, I want you to pull the plug."

"What plug?"

"Now, I'll sing you my favourite song."

A silent rage was boiling inside me. I wanted to push her over onto the floor. I wanted to hurt her. I had been feeling this anger for some time. It was what made me dig my nails into her as I pulled her along, or grab her arm too roughly, or drop her down into a chair with more force than I should have. Sometimes I even thought about not catching her when she stumbled and letting her fall to the ground. As she sang her sad song, my heart heaved with resentment. *Who could be angry at a sick mother? I could.* To make up for my shameful thoughts, I pretended to listen to her. For now at least, pledging promises and pulling plugs were momentarily set aside for singing songs. Suddenly, she grabbed my hands. "My life is over," she cried.

"Dr. DeGroot didn't say you were going to die." I pulled away and flopped onto my side, my back to her.

"Tilda, if I get very bad I want you to do me in," she implored and then looked up at the ceiling as if to beseech the heavens above. "When the time comes, please kill me. It's the only kind thing to do." I looked away and pretended not to hear. "Find a way," she said, and I pretended not to understand.

IT WAS LESS THAN one year later when I came home from school one prematurely dark afternoon to an empty and silent house. The streetlights hummed with electricity in the blue twilight and Christmas lights blinked on the neighbours' trees. I entered the house and moved from room to room, turning on lights as I went. When I got to the kitchen and flicked on the light switch, I found my mother at the table, staring out with blank eyes. I ignored her strange behaviour, opened the refrigerator and stood staring into its depths. "Where's Dad?" I asked casually, mid-bite into an apple.

"In his ivory tower." Then, of all things, she broke into song. "*Spesso vibra per suo gioco, il bendato pargoletto, strali d'oro in umil petto, stral di ferro in nobil seno. Questo manca . . .*"

Scarlatti! Why now the blindfolded boy who pierces a humble breast with golden darts? One victim languishing in vain, while another falls faint? "What's going on?" I yelled. "Where's Dad?"

"The hospital. His heart."

My own heart began pounding wildly. *He's okay*, I told myself. "He's okay," I said out loud to make it so.

"I'll drive," she said with a crazy grin.

She didn't even have a licence, but she got in the driver's seat and somehow we got there.

The doctor said it was a mild heart attack, but my father should take it as a warning.

How strange to see my father lying flat-out in bed, still and quiet, the colour and life drained from him. He propped himself up on one elbow to sip water from a plastic straw bent into a paper cup. A pretty nurse with a swinging ponytail and pink stethoscope around her neck, whose name tag said "Cindy," came in and took my father's pulse with her big, reassuring scuba-diving wristwatch that had dials and buttons on the side. "His vital signs are stable," she told me.

Adopt me, please! I madly radioed her. *Take me home with you. I'll be your little sister.*

My mother and I stayed a few more minutes then kissed him goodnight. When we got off the elevator on the ground floor, she came to an abrupt halt. "Let's stay here in the lobby. My nerves are shot. I need to gather my bearings." She dropped into the nearest chair, and I slumped down low in a chair beside her. My mind wandered off. I was drowsy. . . . She had to gather her bearings . . . *gathering bearings . . . gathering berries in the forest . . . teddy bearings . . . the Bering Strait . . . I will travel far away . . . strawbearings . . . raspbearings.* Sleep was right there behind my eyes. It would be so easy to give in, but I couldn't, I was on duty. *Dr. Ben Casey ordered me to monitor the patient closely. Get him through the night, he'd said. It all depends on you.* I got up and walked around to wake myself up.

"Don't go far," my mother called out, "I may need you."

The Ladies' Auxiliary had set up a little petting zoo for the children in the pediatric ward. There was an aquarium of tropical fish and a tank with a branch upon which an iguana draped itself. A parakeet pecked at its reflection in a little mirror, jabbering "yakkety yakkety yak." I stared deeply into its blue feathers at the back of its neck and in a few seconds I knew what I would do. One day, I would become a real nurse. It made perfect sense. Being a nurse was what I knew best. I liked spending time in hospitals, where problems were solved, grown-ups were in charge, and people knew what they were doing. Pleased with my new plan, I returned to my mother in the lobby.

"If anything happens to your father," she said when she saw me, "promise you'll look after me, that you won't put me away . . . in some *place*."

"Yes, I promise." I took her hand. "Let's go home. Have you found your bearings yet?"

"They're nowhere in sight and I'm worried sick about your father."

One day, when I'm a real nurse, I'll be able to leave at the end of my shift.

3

THEORIZING, CONCEPTUALIZING, AND CATHETERIZING

Over the years, I became very familiar with hospitals. I even grew to love them. In fact, I loved them so much that when I was fourteen, I worked as a candystriper at Toronto General Hospital and spent my summer vacation filling patients' water jugs and delivering flowers and mail. I must have performed my duties well because the next summer I was promoted to the patients' lending library and put in charge of the mobile cart of books and magazines. Most patient rooms had four beds and since there was no air conditioning, the windows were always wide open to let in fresh air and the long, billowing curtains flapped when there was a faint breeze. To the male patients, sitting up in bed, eagerly awaiting my arrival, I handed out dog-eared "spaghetti westerns" by Louis L'Amour and to the women, I gave the purple-prose bodice rippers by authors such as Barbara Cartland and Taylor Caldwell. They were all pleased to see me and to receive light reading material to take their minds off their problems.

In the hospital, I felt at ease, almost happy. I liked watching busy doctors and nurses rushing around with a sense of purpose and importance. And the hospital seemed such an equitable and democratic place. Everyone was in the same boat, dressed in the same flimsy blue hospital gowns and all worried about something. And although it was such a vast, public space, you knew that private, intimate activities were occurring between complete strangers. On any ordinary day, you could see people in various states of distress, crying and moaning, and even though these sights were disturbing, they were fascinating, too. The hospital was a place chock full of mysteries, a repository of intriguing stories. Each patient was a book I wanted to read. Why was that man in the plaid bathrobe sitting in a wheelchair by the window looking so wistful? Why did that woman have a plastic tube sticking out of her nose, and how did it get in there? Why was that old lady tied down in a wheelchair, and why did she keep calling out, "Gladys, Gladys, take me to the bank"? As I walked through the halls, pushing my cart of paperbacks, I imagined that one day I would be a part of it all, a calm and selfless presence ministering to the sick and weary. It didn't seem as if it would be as difficult to take care of strangers as it was taking care of one's family members. I couldn't help my own family, but at least as a nurse I would be able to rescue the rest of the world. Being a nurse would make me a better person.

Best of all, in the hospital, no one knew where I was. I could get lost and not be found. In the basement, there was a chapel and I would often sit in a pew at the back, staring up at the cross above the altar for long periods of time. Other days, I lingered in the hospital gift shop, fingering the pastel knitted booties, pot holders, macramé hanging baskets, and crocheted toilet paper covers (one had a Barbie doll's head and torso sticking out of it) and imagined those sweet grandmothers who must have made them.

By the end of high school, my path was clear. I was desperate to leave home and pragmatic enough to reason that nurses would always be needed. Yes, nursing would be my ticket to ride, my escape route. There were only a few small problems. I had read the Nurse Cherry Ames books and I knew about her porcelain skin, rosy cheeks, and wholesome personality. I knew nurses were still supposed to be angels and heroes. Me? I had more than a touch of the devil. As for opportunities to be heroic, I'd blown those, big time. And weren't nurses supposed to be capable, level-headed, and practical? They were known to be efficient, sensible, and cheerful. I was none of these things, but I would work on myself, I promised. After all, to be a nurse was such an admirable, altruistic thing and how nice it would be to help humanity in some way or another. How good it would feel to be good!

THE FIRST YEAR AT the Faculty of Nursing at the University of Toronto, in 1979, was almost entirely spent in classroom lectures. The required courses were physiology, anatomy, microbiology, biochemistry, and Introduction to Nursing Theory, and for my elective, I chose Feminist Studies. I had every intention of being a diligent student, but all too often I got distracted or was overcome by inertia and stayed home keeping my mother company. When I did make it down to the campus, I usually ended up sitting in a coffee shop with my boyfriend, Larry, and then losing myself altogether for the rest of the afternoon in his parked car to the tune of Marvin Gaye's "Sexual Healing," which we played over and over on his tape deck.* Mind you, a student could sit in those classes, listen to the lectures, write the papers, pass the exams, and never even come near a patient. We only visited the hospital as observers, wearing our navy uniforms and white lab coats, touring the various departments. I wondered where I would eventually work because I didn't have any particular allegiance to a specific organ, such as the heart, which would have led me to cardiology, or the kidneys so I could have chosen nephrology. And I wasn't drawn to the relatively happy obstetrics or orthopedic wards, pediatrics seemed far too daunting, and I couldn't bear to spend much time in the psychiatric wards with its smell of cigarettes, sweat, and despair. The patients there were frightened, angry, or sad, and sometimes all of those things. In truth, it felt too close to home.

---

* Larry was an engineering student I met at one of the campus social events that brought together the mostly all-female nursing class with the mostly all-male engineering class. It was thought important and logical to encourage this traditional pairing, a kind of academic dating service.

During those many hours in the classroom, I sat in the back row with a bag of snacks beside me, watching the professors droning on from the podium. The other nursing students listened intently and took precise notes. I made random scribblings, catching key phrases such as "conceptual framework" or the "theoretical basis of caring." I took notes about how the nurse was to make "therapeutic use of herself" (there was no attempt at gender-equal language as there was no gender equality in nursing) in order to assist "clients"* toward the generally agreed-upon goal of "self-actualization," which was the "achievement of one's full human potential."

Nursing scholars created an entire lingo of "nursing diagnoses," perhaps in order to be like doctors with their "medical diagnoses," and thereby raise our status. For example, "Altered level of comfort" meant pain and "Altered pattern of urinary elimination" was the euphemism for incontinent. "Health maintenance disruption" meant, simply, illness. My personal favourite was "Disordered nutrition; more than body requirements," which meant the patient was overweight.

Sometimes there were debates about what was, in fact, the role of a nurse. They posited a number of theories. One theory was that the nurse was there to assist the patient with self-care and to perform for them what they could not do for themselves. This sounded good to me, but another theory asserted that the nurse's function was to help patients achieve "wellness" and "homeostasis." Another invoked the words of Florence Nightingale: "The nurse is to put the patient in the condition for Nature to do the work of healing." Another position claimed the nurse was a "body expert" and "health counsellor." Oh, there were nursing theories aplenty, oodles of them!

I think the professors felt they had to justify nursing as a profession worthy of university study. After all, for years, most nurses had diplomas and learned on the job, working in hospitals. One professor insisted that the rightful place of nursing was at the

---

* The term "patient" was considered paternalistic, yet I noticed that real nurses and doctors called them patients.

"Table of the Humanities," in that it drew from the disciplines of philosophy, sociology, and psychology. Another argued that nursing straddled an equally secure position at the "Table of the Sciences." Regrettably, I raised my hand to ask, "Doesn't nursing also have a place at the *Kitchen Table*?" The professor frowned, but I felt that to be a nurse required certain personal, human qualities such as courtesy, warmth, kindness, and respect, attributes one presumably learned at home. No, they countered. These old-fashioned values held nursing back from making progress. Clinging to these outdated notions kept nursing in the Dark Ages. To be a nurse required skill and knowledge, not merely virtue and morality.

But if nursing was both a science and an art, the science – the math and chemistry, etc. – was the easy part. The "art" involved lofty goals that were difficult, if not impossible, to attain. It was the "art" of nursing that required the nurse to enter the patient's world, to understand the patient's point of view and mitigate his isolation or her suffering. As a nurse, you were there to understand your patients' existential questions and to assuage their pain, whether of body, mind, or spirit. You were expected to receive without judgment their emotional expression, whether it was to cry or to complain, or even to be rude to you. You were to praise them when they passed gas after surgery or had a successful bowel movement and then go off and empty the bedpan cheerfully. Your only need was to be needed and to meet other people's needs. If a patient rang the call bell, you were to jump. You were there to make a cup of tea, if required. Along with all of that and above all, you were to assist your patient to achieve the ultimate, un-contested goal of all human beings: self-actualization. Oh yes, and don't forget about their medications, fluid balances (their "in's and out's"), IVs, dressings, plus all the secretarial work, too. It was a tall order. No wonder they called us angels.

IT WASN'T UNTIL second year that they finally let us get our hands on real, live "clients." My first one was Mrs. Lenore Thompson, an eighty-three-year-old woman living in a retirement home in downtown Toronto. (I had to chuckle when I noticed that the facility was located kitty corner to The Anti-Aging Store, a place that sold elixirs, balms, and potions, touted to be life-enhancing and prolonging.) I was supposed to interview her and identify any health problems. She was a regal, white-haired lady who opened her display case to show me her collection of glass unicorns with great pride. She brought out her blood-pressure pills and I made a note of their names and the dosages she was taking. Then, she invited me to join her for lunch in the communal dining room. She cut up a slice of pizza with her knife and fork and chewed slowly. Then she put two chocolate sundaes on a tray and asked me to carry it back to her room. We sat enjoying them, but then it was time for "business" and my hands suddenly got jittery when I asked if I could take her vital signs.

"Do you promise to return them to me afterwards?" she said impishly.

That morning, I had made sure to put on my watch that had a second hand so I would be able to take my patient's pulse. It was eighty beats per minute, strong and steady. (I had taken mine earlier and it was right up there, racing at 122.) Her blood pressure was high at 160 over 95, but she promised to cut back on her sodium intake. I looked at the thermometer and hesitated. Should I tell her that she was extremely hypothermic? Her temperature was so low it barely registered! I broke the news to her.

"Perhaps it's because of the ice cream, dear?" she asked helpfully.

"Ah, yes. Of course." It reminded me of those myths of patients who prolonged their hospital stay by putting a thermometer in their mouth after drinking a hot beverage to simulate a fever.

Next, from the corner of my eye, without letting on what I was doing, I counted her respirations so that she would not speed them up or slow them down to confound me, as I'd heard that some patients did.

"You're a nice girl, dearie," she said, catching me watching her chest rise and fall. "You've a sweet face."

"Thank you," I said, but inside I cringed, thinking of my mother. *You're wrong there, lady. I'm neither nice nor sweet.*

EVERY MORNING, before leaving for my classes, I put out my mother's pills for the day and made sure there were plenty of the small brown glass bottles filled with my father's tiny white nitro-glycerin pills for chest pain. "Make sure they're with him at all times," his doctor had instructed me. "His life depends upon it." My father claimed it was nothing but a sugar pill, but the label said *sublingual tablet, indicated for fast-acting vasodilation of the coronary arteries.* I put a bottle in the glove compartment in his car, one next to his typewriter, and one on the spice rack in between the marjoram and the oregano. He popped a few of those pills when he would pull up short on winter evenings and his face went ashen as he set out for his university classes in pre-Confederation history or art appreciation. Then he could carry on like an Arctic explorer, his breath frosty in the air and snow crunching under his feet.

When I came home from school, I fed my mother and got her ready for bed. Sometimes, I claimed to have a lot of schoolwork and let my father take over. Once, after putting her to bed, he joined me with his crossword puzzle and settled in front of the TV. "How do *you* do it?" I asked him.

"I love her," he said simply. "Hey, Til, what's a four-letter word for a Mexican pot?"

It was all he had to say on that matter, yet about everything else he spoke endlessly.

"IT WILL BE A powerful experience," said students in my Feminist Studies class, encouraging me to join them on a march for International Women's Day. We had been learning about the history of women's oppression by the male patriarchy, about the Women's Liberation movement, and useful things such as "assertiveness training" and "consciousness-raising." "There'll be thousands of women marching in solidarity," they said. "Don't miss it." On a blustery day in March, I joined those women and some men, as we started on Queen Street and marched up Spadina Avenue, our arms linked. There were women of all colours, lesbians, straight, liberals, socialists, macrobiotics and vegans; professors, filmmakers, and abortion activists; women with babies on their backs, with children in hand. We wore buttons on our jean jackets that said: "Sisterhood Is Powerful," and "Women Make Policy, Not Coffee." "Take back the night," we chanted. "Women's right, women's might!"

How thrilling it felt to belong! At the end of the march we hugged each other and pledged to keep up the good fight. I decided to stop off at a Kensington Market *groceria* to call my friend Joy on a pay phone. We were making dinner and our boyfriends were coming over that evening, and I wanted to find out if we needed anything. She picked up on the first ring. "Phone your brother," she said. "Right away."

"What for?" I said, ignoring the urgency in her voice.

"Just do it, now."

So I did.

"I've got some bad news." Stephen tried to soften his curt tone. "Are you sitting down?"

Like they say in the movies. Maybe this is a movie.

"I don't know how to say this . . ."

It was strange to hear a member of my family at a loss for words . . .

"Dad died."

I held the phone away and tried to imagine my father gone. Impossible! My brother's voice continued on, like the barking of a dog in the distance. I put the phone down with shaking hands and stumbled along the sawdust-strewn grocery aisles, toward the exit. Seeing my distress, the worried owner hurried after me but I waved him off and ran out into the cool air. The market was closing for the day. The vendors were putting away their baskets of fruits and vegetables, tubs of cheese, and bins of rice and grains. I ran through the grey slush in the streets as tears streamed down my face.

I CAN HARDLY REMEMBER the funeral, I was in shock and pre-occupied with holding my mother together and upright. Afterwards, I brought my mother home, and it was just the two of us. Now, I was in charge of everything. I put out her slippers and nightgown and went to get her ready for bed. The problem was, she was nowhere to be found. I searched the house, calling her name, but either she had wandered away or was playing a twisted game of hide-and-go-seek. At last, I found her in the base-ment, standing next to the furnace, shifting from foot to foot. I pulled her along up the stairs and tugged her nightgown down over her head. I shoved her feet into her terrycloth slippers and didn't even bother brushing her teeth. I placed her pills on her tongue, held a glass of water to her lips, and waited impatiently. They stuck there melting. "Swallow them!" I shouted at her. *Do I have to do that for you, too?*

"How do I know you're not trying to poison me?" she asked with a demure smile.

Could she read my mind? If so, she would know that I wasn't planning to kill her, but I would have preferred her dead instead of my father. I hated myself for my wicked thoughts. As I eased her down onto the toilet seat and handed her a wad of paper, I prayed she would wipe herself. She sat giggling. "It won't come out."

I looked away to give her privacy. At my tragic clown face in the mirror, I burst out laughing, a vicious, pathetic laughter. *How could my father do this to me?* I was furious, but cackled with laughter even more. I went to put away my mother's clothes and turn down her covers, but when I came back, she was gone again. "Where are you?" I dashed from room to room and noticed the open front door. I ran outside and found her sitting behind the wheel of the car in the driveway. She turned the key in the ignition and the engine started up. "Mother, please come inside. It's late. It's cold." She shifted into reverse. I opened the car door, but with surprising force she pulled it shut and released the hand brake. "Let me come with you." I dashed around to the passenger side, climbed in, and just before she drove off I lunged for the keys and turned off the igni-tion. "Come back into the house," I begged.

"Your father is at the subway station. I have to pick him up."

"Mother," I said, taking her hand, "I'm sorry to have to tell you, but he died."

"Don't you *do re mi* me, like all the rest."

"Come back into the house. It's time for bed."

"Do you have any understanding of what's going on?" She leaned on me as we walked back in.

"Very little," I admitted.

"You know what?" She brightened with a plan. "I'm going to do what I'm going to do and afterwards, I'll tell you what I've done."

"Good idea." I trudged up the stairs, guiding her up in front of me. I couldn't wait to get into bed and escape behind my closed eyes. But sometime during the night she stood over me, shaking me awake. "Where's the conductor? Who's keeping the beat? The soloist is waiting."

"What are you talking about?" I mumbled.

"I need to see samples of organisms. I have certain stipulations."

"Go back to sleep, it's too early to get up." I rolled over but somewhere between sleep and morning, I heard her say, "I called the fire department and the police." Next thing I knew, sirens wailed down the street toward our house.

I TRIED TO GET back to my classes at the university, but I noticed that wherever I left my mother in the morning was where I usually found her when I returned home at the end of the day. One evening she pointed in an agitated manner at an empty chair and said, "Does that man come here every day?"

"Who are you talking to?" I barked at her, like a policeman to a suspected criminal.

"*Salut!*" She clinked an imaginary glass at her imaginary companion. "Leave us alone."

"Mother, do you know where you are?" I said wearily.

"Pay the driver and give me my change!"

Suddenly, I could see what was about to happen and I rushed over to her but it was too late. A dark wet puddle was spreading around her on the velvet chair, dripping down and onto the carpet. I pulled her out of the chair, dragged her along to her bedroom, put a diaper on her, and we both fell asleep.

"Severe cognitive impairment can occur after a psychological shock such as a sudden loss," Dr. DeGroot explained when I called to tell her what was happening. "It's a mild psychosis or a traumatic disorientation. It sounds like she's pleasantly confused. How's she managing with her ADL?"

Oh, those darn Activities of Daily Living! The very things that had always been so difficult for her: walking, talking, bathing, eating, and getting dressed. "With my help . . . ," I told the doctor and as I got off the phone, I sat there considering my own ADL of late: mulling, pondering, worrying, stewing, and wondering. I longed to lie in bed and sob for hours, but it was a luxury I couldn't afford. I got up, got myself dressed, then my mother, poured cornflakes into a bowl, lifted spoonfuls to her mouth, eased her in and out of chairs, and then sat down to contemplate my life of servitude. I saw everything through a soft, fuzzy film of tears that I didn't even wipe away. Why bother? More came. Tiny pulses of energy kept me going, but at times I gave up and joined my mother as we sat in our nightgowns watching game shows and evangelical healers on the television.

"What have you been up to?" Joy called to ask. "My mother is very worried about you."

"We get up. We watch *The Friendly Giant* and *The Price Is Right*."

Joy's mother, Bunny, got on the phone. "Tilda dear, you have to get some help. Ask your brothers if you can afford to hire someone to help you."

"I promised her I'd always take care of her." *But that was a long time ago, wasn't it? It's a promise I can no longer keep.*

"It's too much for you on your own," Bunny insisted.

My brother Stephen had taken over managing the finances and had been giving me money for groceries and medications. He told me that there were sufficient funds to hire a caregiver for my mother and so I called the Loving Care Agency (because of the name) and hired a Personal Support Worker. I had to avert my eyes from my mother's accusatory glare when Pearl Bernard arrived, but Pearl soon won her over. And when she put her strong arms around me, I shivered at her warm touch. "You must have loved your dear father," she said. Tears sprung to my eyes. Yes, I did, but only now that he was gone did I realize just how much. Yes, I loved him, but I hadn't shown it and had never told him. Too often, I had been irritated and impatient at his corny jokes. I had refused his exotic meals and hadn't played along with his word games or puzzles.

Pearl prepared hearty foods like Callaloo soup, salt fish, and mashed plantains, and my mother quickly regained her appetite. I went shopping for a pair of orthopedic shoes, a raised toilet seat and railing, and finally, with Pearl's gentle persuasion, the wheelchair my mother had resisted for so long. Grief had brought me to a standstill. My life had been shutting down, but Pearl got us all going again. I even returned to my classes, and the professors and other students all helped me ease back in. Thanks to Pearl, a nurse in her own right, I managed to finish my third year at university.

In my fourth and final year, we had lots of clinical work in the hospital with real patients, always under the supervision of a registered nurse. Most RNs didn't mind and a few actually welcomed it, but there were always one or two who didn't like it at all.

"It's not an option. It's part of your job description," I heard the manager tell Joan, one of the nurses assigned to supervise me and who didn't look too happy about it. She was heavy-set and wore clunky white Swedish clogs and made a face as soon as she saw the knapsack I was lugging around, practically split open from the heavy textbooks I was carrying. (I had taken pains to ensure that the university insignia emblazoned on it was hidden from view as I had begun to sense that this was a point of contention.)

"What've you got in there?" she asked.

"Books," I muttered.

"Well, you won't be needing any of those around here. You become an RN, a Real Nurse, on the job, taking care of patients. Not from reading books."

I apologized and trotted after her down the hall. "Tilda? What kind of name is that? Is it short for something?" Joan asked, not looking back. "Where'd you get a name like that?"

"My parents had a sense of humour."

Joan was gruff and a bit rough around the edges, but she was gentle and kind toward patients and I learned a lot from her. She inspired confidence by the smooth way she did technical tasks, all the while comforting her patients with a kind word or touch of her hand. We had six patients to take care of that day, but the first priority was an elderly lady whose fluid balance was uncertain. "Let's see you go in there and put a catheter in this lady," she said, standing outside the patient's room. "Her urine output has dropped off and we need to follow her fluid balance more closely." She handed me an armful of supplies. I stood there contemplating the task at hand and realized that although I knew how to theorize and conceptualize, I did not know how to catheterize. Joan took one look at me and chuckled as she took back the supplies. "Come on," she said kindly, "watch me." She led the way and I followed in after her. First, Joan explained to the patient what we were going to do. "I'm going to clean you down there," she said to her as she closed the curtains around the bed and gently uncovered her naked white thighs. Joan ended up letting me do the procedure with her close guidance. It was tricky, as you had to keep a strictly sterile field in order to prevent introducing bacteria, but I managed it successfully. When I told Joy about it later, she thought it a strange thing to take pleasure in, but my fellow nursing students understood exactly how incredibly satisfying it was to see the stream of urine fill the tube once I had positioned it correctly and secured it in the patient's bladder.

We were busy that day. Joan and I discharged two patients and received two more from the ICU. I thought I was doing pretty well under Joan's close watch, but later that day, in the nurses' station, as I stood behind a floor-to-ceiling rack of patient charts, I was mortified to hear her and another nurse on the other side of the rack complaining and making fun of the students. I heard Joan's voice first.

"The patient has Alzheimer's but she didn't seem to pick up on that. I found the two of them in the lounge, watching an old *Beverly Hillbillies* rerun."

That would be me. It was the episode where Ellie Mae Clampitt's pet chicken and a rooster stood at a miniature grand piano, pecking out a duet. Who could resist that one?

". . . they were sitting there, laughing their heads off and my student didn't even notice the patient's nasal prongs had slipped out of her nose and she wasn't getting her oxygen."

"You think *your* student is bad," the other nurse said with a sigh. "Mine gave her patient's meds through the naso-gastric tube and then reconnected it to the drainage system so it all drained out – can you believe it? Then she set up a basin for her patient's morning care with only an inch of lukewarm water in it. What are they teaching these university students?"

"Mine's useless, too." Another nurse must have joined the conversation. "She accidentally threw a patient's bathrobe into the dirty laundry bin, so I sent her down to the basement to go through all the dirty linen to find it."

"And have you seen how these *university* nurses make a bed?" Joan asked. "When I was training, the head nurse stood at the door and checked that the fold of the sheets was facing out, not the open edges. Those were the days of real nursing. I'm telling you, I don't know what's wrong with this generation of nurses. They haven't a clue."

Our professors had warned us about bully nurses who "eat their young." Nurses were part of an "oppressed group," they had explained, and as such, often resorted to "lateral aggression" in order to raise their status in the hospital hierarchy. Of all those nursing theories I had studied, I was beginning to sense that what I would need most to survive as a nurse was Darwin's Theory of Evolution – "survival of the fittest"! This was part of the initiation rites, to be sure, but I couldn't disagree with what they were saying.

I would be scared to have me for a nurse. But I suppose I was a good enough nurse.

At times, I struggled with what it meant to be a nurse. Sometimes you had to take charge of situations or impose your will on patients, and I found that difficult. For example, if a patient refused to get up out of bed right after surgery, I didn't like having to nag them about it, even though it was necessary for their breathing and circulation. If they didn't do what we said or wouldn't take their meds, we were supposed to record that they were uncooperative or noncompliant. Many aspects of being a nurse involved policing and enforcement, and I was uncomfortable in that role. And so often, a nurse had to inflict discomfort in order to be of help. I flinched more than my patients did when I gave an injection or pulled off the tape around an IV. There was so much to do, so many important details to remember, and everything was to be documented because it was drilled into us that "not charted, not done."

But there was so much I *did* like, especially wearing my uniform and being part of the team. I liked to fill my pockets with what I saw real nurses carry: different types of tape, bandage scissors, a clamp, and medication labels. I liked caring for fresh post-operative patients. They were cool and clammy with an anaesthetic-induced grey pallor, and when I put warmed flannel sheets on them, they woke up grateful, not only to have survived the operation, but for my being their nurse. I liked bathing patients and I didn't mind emptying bedpans of urine, though I couldn't bring myself to touch people's slimy false teeth without gagging. And I liked how the nurse's presence was constant and sustained, whereas the doctors' visits were brief and intermittent. Nurses talked in a casual, familiar way to patients, especially compared to the formal, reserved manner in which the doctors spoke. They had no airs or pretensions and I liked that.

AS GRADUATION NEARED, everyone was excited about landing jobs and getting started on our careers. We had a lot to live up to. High goals had been set for us. We were warned that we might at first

experience a temporary period of "reality shock" when we actually entered the work world, but not to worry, in no time at all, we
would adjust. We *had* to adjust. After all, we were to be the
"change agents" of the future, they told us, the ones who would
bring nursing into the twenty-first century and save the health-care
system. I wanted to do all of that, of course, but in the meantime,
I was just praying that I wouldn't give someone the wrong pills or
miss a serious sign that indicated danger.

"MOTHER," I SAID to her one evening, on Pearl's day off, "let's go
out, you and me. I want to talk with you about something."

"I don't want to go anywhere. I want to go somewhere," she
said in her muddled way, but I got her into the car and drove to
Fran's Restaurant, where they were having a "Festival of Raisins":
Raisin Pie, Raisin Cake, and Raisin Pudding. *Raison d'être* was
what I needed. "Mother, I have something important to tell you."

"How thrilling," she said, rolling her eyes.

"When I graduate in June, I want to go to Israel. I've heard they
need nurses there and I want to see the country and travel. Pearl
will take care of you."

"In my heyday, you were a mere essence." She giggled. "I'm
getting a surge of Genevieve."

Frustration rose up at the back of my throat, tasting of acid.
How could she segue in and out of insanity? "Are you trying to
drive me crazy?" I stood up to go.

"Go practise your part in the play," she muttered and beat a
retreat behind her eyes.

When we got home, she exploded with a secret source of energy
just like that day when she destroyed her records. She began
frantically rummaging through drawers and closets looking for
something. She bent down to pluck at invisible objects on the floor.
"Something about you disturbs me," she fretted. "You have an
abnormal mental make-up and smell like polka dots. Your words
come from a garbage can and those men you brought home
damaged Pearl. I won't stand for it."

"What men?"

"Switch over your switches and you'll see them!" She grabbed my sleeve and dropped to her *sotto voce*, hushed, yet powerful enough for the audience in the back row. Suddenly, something frightened her. "Listen!" she cried, "Pearl is having a seizure! Go help her." Pearl, back from her day off, was singing "Abide With Me" as she ran my mother's bath. "Pearl's fine, don't worry," I said. "You're torturing my central nervous system," she said as I handed her over to Pearl. I picked up the phone to buy a ticket to Tel Aviv.

THE DAY BEFORE my flight, I sat down for one last run-through of the "reality orientation" exercises Dr. DeGroot had taught me. "Mother, listen up." I pulled her chin to face me. "You are Elinor Shalof. It is 1983. You live in Toronto. Pearl is taking care of you. I'm sorry to have to tell you, but your husband, my father, unfortunately –"

"There, there," Pearl cut in.

"That's your version." My mother sat still, smug with her truth.

"Well, what's yours?"

"Oranges and lemons."

"Sometimes she get mixed up, but she know what's what. She do!" Pearl said as she smoothed my mother's dark, wavy hair and wiped her mouth. She had a knack for making her look glamorous. "She good enough, man. Good enough, I say!"

"She's going downhill," I grumbled.

"Maybe, but oh Lord, what a voice she have! She open the mouth and out it comes. Glorious! Some voices you have to listen for a while until you hear them. This voice you hear right away. I would do anything for that woman!"

The next morning, my mother stood in front of the door, frozen and rooted in place. Her nylon stockings drooped, and she gripped the floor with her toes for balance. "Don't go," she said, and tried to stamp her foot. Pearl explained it to me. "Your mother, she want what's best for you. She do. Put your questions to God. Place your faith in Him. Ask Him for a sign."

"What kind of sign?"

"Open the Book to any page and there you will see the light and the way." She handed me a brand new, white, leather-bound Bible and I slipped it into my knapsack alongside a *People* magazine with an article about Princess Diana and her post-partum blues, to read on the airplane. "See God's purposes, Romans 8:28, and God's wise plan in Corinthians 2:9."

I hugged her. I took comfort wherever I could find it and even though we were Jewish, I was beginning to prefer Pearl's understanding of things.

"I'm a grown-up, I want you to know." My mother swayed from side to side.

"Who said you weren't?"

She shifted from one foot to the other. "So why do you put me in that baby carriage?" She pointed to the wheelchair parked at the front door.

"Let us offer up a prayer," Pearl interjected, standing beside her. My mother leaned into her as they bowed their heads. "May the Almighty bless and keep our dear Tilda safe in His loving care. May she go with the love and mercy of our Lord and Saviour, Jesus Christ. Amen." She walked me to the front door and I stood there, flanked by two duffel bags. I steeled myself not to cry, not now.

"Stay," my mother said, "you promised you wouldn't leave me."

Pearl opened the door. "Don't worry, dear. I'll take care of your mom. It's okay." She pushed me forward with her hand on my shoulder. "Go now," she said, setting me free.

I took one last look back and then went.

4

ICE CREAM DAYS

On my own, high in the sky, enveloped by the gentle roar of the airplane's engines, I was calm. I had no idea where I was going, where I'd stay or find work, but I was thrilled at the prospect of my adventure. Yes, I was finally a Real Nurse and now had the documents to prove it. However, even with my university degree there were no jobs for nurses in Canada. It was the downward swing of the boom-bust economic cycle, and as hospitals downsized, nurses were the first to be cut. I wasn't worried because I had long ago decided on my plans upon graduation. I would go to Israel. I told everyone I wanted to connect with my Jewish identity. This was true enough, but I kept quiet about my other reasons: I was seeking fun, romance, and danger!

ELEVEN YEARS BEFORE, at the age of thirteen, I had travelled to Israel with my father. He had wanted to expand my horizons and believed that Israel was the place to start. That was back in 1972, in the heady, jubilant years after the Six-Day War and prior to the devastating Yom Kippur War, in which Israel was attacked and its very survival threatened. Then, in 1976, there was Israel's courageous rescue of kidnapped hostages in Entebbe, and in 1991, the daring and precise attack on Iraq's nuclear reactor. Of course, books influenced me too, especially *Exodus*, by Leon Uris (a very hunky Paul Newman starred in the movie version) and *Raquela, Woman of Israel*, about a beautiful and dedicated nurse who rescued lots of sweaty soldiers wounded on the battlefield. She nursed them back to life and they all fell in love with her.

Something happened on that trip with my father that drew me inexorably back to Israel. It was a small thing, but the memory of it stayed with me. It happened as we were getting ready to leave. I stood on the hot tarmac about to make my way up the metal staircase of the El Al flight to return home to Canada. Soldiers in khaki uniforms surrounded the plane, guarding it as they did every aircraft that flew in and out of Israel. One particularly stunning, suntanned soldier, his rifle slung casually across his back looked right at me and flashed me a slow, knowing wink. *Come back*, that wink said, and I knew then and there that I would one day.

This time, arriving in Israel, I felt an immediate sense of belonging to the country and its history even though I knew no one and barely spoke the language. From the airport, I took a bus to the nearest hospital, called Tel HaShomer, a large medical centre located beside a military base just outside of Tel Aviv. It was early summer and the windows were wide open on the bus. I smelled a beautiful, sweet aroma and inhaled deeply. I guess I must have had "tourist" written all over me because the passenger sitting beside me pointed to the orchard groves lining the road. "Orange blossoms," he said. "Welcome to Israel."

At the hospital, I met the Director of Nursing, Shoshana Zamir, a tall, commanding woman in a white uniform and sandals. She welcomed me warmly like I was her long-lost daughter and praised my halting Hebrew. It was as if by clasping me to her huge bosom, she was enfolding me into the entire country, its history and collective destiny. Yes, indeed, they needed nurses badly, she lamented, especially well-educated ones like me. There was a shortage of nurses in Israel and an over-abundance of doctors. "I guess every Jewish mother wants her son to be a doctor," Shoshana said with a chuckle, "and not many Jewish mothers encourage their daughters to be nurses, do they?"

Nor their sons either, I thought. But surely it was only a matter of time until gender equality would be achieved in the nursing profession?

Shoshana suggested I start in a general medicine ward where most of the patients were elderly, bedridden, and had chronic illnesses with no cure. It wasn't the most exciting department, especially for a nurse with my impressive credentials, she said, but she wanted me to share with those nurses the benefit of my university education and thereby raise the standards of the nursing care. She walked me over to the patient wards, which were actually rows of Quonset huts, long, narrow buildings that had been built, makeshift, in the 1940s. They were made of corrugated steel and were so rundown it looked like they should be condemned. But as shabby and ramshackle as they were on the outside, they were gleaming and modern on the inside, replete with the unmistakable smells of disinfectant, rubbing alcohol, fresh laundry, and urine underlying it all.

Shoshana introduced me to Yaffa, the head nurse, who had a roly-poly body, solid as a truck, encased in a crisp white uniform. Sticking straight up on her head was a white winged cap, its corner points sharp as daggers. "Teelda? What kind of name is zat?" Yaffa made my name sound too much like the word *gleeda*, which was Hebrew for ice cream. She looked me over. "Where's your *kep*?"

"I don't have one," I answered with a superior smile. Obviously, Yaffa was not aware of the great strides being made in our profession. The nurses' cap was an outdated symbol of a long-gone time when nurses were passive, subordinate, and merely doctors' assistants. "Nurses don't wear caps any more. They're old-fashioned."

"You're not a nurse without zee kep. Wear it tomorrow if you want to work here."

Well, we'll see about that, I thought.

"Vhat? Again vit no kep?" Yaffa said as soon as she saw me the next morning. (She insisted on speaking to me in English, even though my broken Hebrew was better than her broken English.)

"Affirmative," I replied in an English I knew she wouldn't be able to grasp, "I refuse to don the aforementioned distasteful article of obsolete headgear."

"You are forbidden to take care of patients without zee kep." Yaffa folded her arms across her chest. I stood equally firm. She handed me a mop and a pail. "Here," she said. "Do *sponja*."

I lasted two weeks, hating every minute of it. Every morning I did the *sponja*. It involved filling a bucket with warm soapy water, dumping it out all over the floor, and then sweeping the water outside into the cow pasture behind the hut. Afterwards, I folded laundry and gave out lunch trays to the patients. The other nurses under Yaffa's regime tiptoed around her. She scolded them if they so much as made a sound during the doctors' rounds. It was demoralizing. This wasn't nursing! Luckily, Shoshana Zamir came for a visit and saw how miserable I was. I guess she didn't want to lose me, as she offered me a position in a new unit to be added onto the back of Barrack Thirty-six, to be called Thirty-six Alef, which tacked on the first letter of the Hebrew alphabet.

"It will be a bone marrow transplant unit. You will start working in the hematology clinic and when the transplant unit is opened, you'll work there. They've pioneered this procedure in Seattle, San Francisco, and Jerusalem, and now we'll be on the map, too. How does that sound?" Hematology was blood diseases and that meant mostly cancers, like leukemia and lymphoma. It was an honour to be chosen for the challenge; Shoshana must have seen potential in me.

After I'd been in Israel a few weeks, I called home. My mother was the same: angry, confused, and inaudible. Pearl seemed to be managing just fine. Once again, I thanked her for making it possible for me to have my freedom. I had even made progress toward my other goal – to let loose and have fun. I had begun to make friends with the other nurses and doctors. On days off they took me to interesting places, like caves with stalagmites and stalactites, a Tel Aviv discotheque, a place on the West Bank called "Little Switzerland" because of its lush valleys and hills, and of course "up" to Jerusalem, the city holy to so many. The language actually dictated that one "ascended to Jerusalem," and I understood that the grammar referred not only to the elevation above sea level, but to the spiritual high possible there.

Even with the tensions and ever-present threat of war, it was easy to find fun in Israel. Sometimes, even my bus ride home after work provided unexpected delights. One night after finishing a shift well after midnight, the driver serenaded the passengers with folk songs as he detoured off the main road to take me right to my apartment door to ensure I got home safely. On another chilly and rainy night, I sat at the back of the bus. "Do you want to get warm?" a handsome soldier asked and opened his jacket for me to snuggle up close. We stayed on long past our stops, quietly making out in the shadows.

It didn't take long before I was conversing in basic Hebrew. I had never learned it as a colloquial language, only as it was written in prayer books. The modern vernacular was vibrant, colourful, and at times, unavoidably blunt. It simply did not allow one to sit on the fence, beat around the bush, or act false. In Hebrew, I spoke louder and more boldly and found myself saying things I would never have dared say in English. Perhaps it was also because in Israel, I had a fresh start. People only knew me as I was then, in front of them, during that blossoming time of my life. And when I spoke to men in Hebrew, I felt beautiful and alive. It was as if sexual innuendo was built right into the grammar. The different forms of address identified the speaker and the one spoken to as male or female. It was a turn-on when a man recognized my femininity by the suffixes he used. When I spoke, I identified myself as a woman and him as a man. I'm not sure this titillating *frisson* was what ancient biblical linguists intended, but that was how I experienced it.

The hematology outpatient clinic was a casual, informal place, despite the seriousness of the patients' illnesses. The doctors and nurses all wore loose green scrubs and sandals, and everyone called each other by their first names. Every patient had to have blood tests before seeing the doctor. Aviva Shofet was one of the senior nurses in the clinic and she taught me how to draw blood and start IVs and soon I got pretty good at it. It was a thrill to see the tiny speck of blood, called the "flashback," in the plastic sheath of the angiocath. It was the surest sign I was in the vein. I discovered that the best way to locate a "difficult vein" was by touch and sometimes I even closed my eyes to feel for it. I learned the secret, idiosyncratic places in patients' arms and hands where the best veins were hidden. First I got to know a patient's veins, and then I got to know the patient.

One day an entire platoon of new soldiers came to the clinic. They weren't sick, but they needed routine blood tests before Basic Training. That day I palpated hundreds of "antecubital spaces" – the soft place inside the bend in the arm – where easy, obvious veins are often found. One soldier boasted how tough he was, that he had seen it all, but he cringed when I drew his blood and looked like he was about to faint. He could take everything, he claimed – except the sight of blood.

Aviva drew my attention to a number circled on one soldier's chart. It was his medical profile, she explained, but even the most virile, healthy-looking male specimens could only achieve a ninety-seven out of one hundred. "They can never get one hundred. Do you know why?" she asked with a grin, knowing that I did not. "They're all circumcised, which is a surgical procedure, so they get three points knocked off the top – so to speak – right away."

Children, even infants, were brought to that clinic, and Aviva explained that if they were upset and crying, it was actually the best time to swiftly slip in a needle because their veins bulged out and were easier to visualize. So, when tiny baby Adi, who was just six months old, was brought in to the clinic screaming in her mother's arms, I gritted my teeth, steeled myself, and nailed that vein, as slender as a single silken thread. Aviva nodded her approval. *Here I am, taking care of kids with cancer*, I praised myself. *See, my mind can trump my emotions when necessary.*

After they had their blood drawn, the patients waited to see the doctor, who would examine them and review the results of those tests. Meanwhile, the nurses began the treatments that usually involved chemotherapy, antibiotics, and/or blood transfusions. An astonishing array of patients came to us in that tiny clinic.

A Bedouin shepherd arrived for his chemotherapy, directly from tending his sheep. He had dark skin and a bushy white moustache that curled up at the ends. He wore the traditional *keffiyah* wrapped around his head and rested his walking stick made from the branch of an olive tree against the wall. As he sat down, ancient dust and biblical sand billowed up from the folds of his caftan. When I looked out the window, I identified his "vehicle": tied to a post in the parking lot was a donkey swishing its tail.

A cultured Romanian woman was nervous. Her veins were deep in her fleshy arms, but I managed to find a tiny blue one, hidden on the inner aspect of her pale forearm. When she smiled weakly in thanks to me, I noticed her bleeding gums and I knew I would likely be transfusing her with platelets later that day.

Twenty-one-year-old Talia had completed her army service and had just been accepted to law school, but on a hiking trip in the Galilee with friends, after climbing Mount Gilboa, she had noticed bruises along her arms and legs. She was diagnosed with a rare disease called aplastic anemia, a complete malfunction of the bone marrow and only a transplant could save her life. Luckily, her sister was a close and willing match.

Amos was a brilliant scientist, specializing in cellular biology, who was diagnosed with leukemia. I asked him what it was like to know so much about his disease, right down to the molecular level. "I wish I didn't know," he said bitterly. "I can't enjoy the luxury of denial."

Dr. Yosef Ben Cassis, the Chief of Hematology, grabbed his shoulders and shook him lightly. "But, Amos, you have the best diagnosis," he said. "You of all people should realize that! Your type of leukemia has the best survival rate. Don't you realize how lucky you are?"

No, he didn't. Apparently, he didn't want any kind of leukemia.

Samuel Abulafia always came with his wife who fussed over him. He was a well-dressed, elegant gentleman who whistled to the little sparrows outside the clinic. He had pet names for them such as "Tzippy," "Pastilla," or "Yona," and they would alight upon his shoulder, come right into the clinic with him, and keep him company during his chemotherapy.

There was Yeshai, a young rabbinical student, dressed in a long black coat and black hat. He was pale, not just from leukemia, but from living a life indoors, immersed in the study of the Torah and its commentaries, the Talmud. His strict religious observance prohibited a woman's touch, except in cases of "life endangerment." So, when I held his arm to take blood from him, I teased him by reminding him it was for medical reasons only, but I couldn't coax a smile out of him. One day, as he lay on a stretcher receiving his chemo, I asked him about the tract he was studying. It concerned the question of whether or not it was permissible to eat an egg laid on the Sabbath.

"But the chicken did the work," I said, getting involved in a discussion I knew nothing about.

"Are Jewish chickens supposed to observe the Sabbath, too?" the patient lying in the bed next to Yeshai joined in. He was a secular Jew, a farmer from a kibbutz.

"It is forbidden," Yeshai began weakly. His chemo was finished and I opened up his saline line to give him more fluids. He was shivering and I covered him with a wool blanket. "It is forbidden to partake of products created on the Sabbath. The chicken has broken the sanctity of the Sabbath and thus the egg it produced is rendered unkosher."

"We must train our Jewish chickens better," the farmer said, bemused.

Yuri was an eighteen-year-old new immigrant who had had to defer his army duty because of his illness. He was worried about the stigma of not serving in the army, but I heard Dr. Ben Cassis say privately that he would probably not survive long enough to experience that stigma and would have to endure only the stigma of cancer. His parents tiptoed around him, speaking in Russian. Yuri translated for them and had his own questions, too, such as, "What does 'white blood cell' mean?" or "When will be my last day?" He was alarmed to overhear Dr. Ben Cassis say he had "no cells." He came over to where I stood in the blood-drawing alcove. "What that means, no cells?" I explained that the chemotherapy had wiped out all his cells, good and bad, to the lowest possible level, called the nadir. This had made him very vulnerable to infection, I said, but soon his bone marrow would begin to produce healthy cells that would protect him.

Later, Aviva reprimanded me. "Don't talk to patients so much, Tilda. Leave that to the doctor." But Hannah, who was the head nurse of the clinic, didn't mind what I did and she preferred to offer patients warmth and affection rather than factual information. She was a petite, lively woman with a mane of wild dark blond hair and lots of jangling jewellery and silver rings on her fingers. Hannah ran the clinic like the hostess of a cocktail lounge, moving amongst the patients, chatting and laughing with families, offering advice, tea and coffee, and ensuring everyone was comfy. She made her rounds to each patient receiving chemo or a transfusion, offered blankets (it was blazing hot, but after chemo, most patients felt chilled), painkillers, or a clean vomit basin, and always a kind, encouraging word.

"*Yeyiyeh tov*," it'll be good, or "*Ha kol besder*," everything's all right, she said to Israeli patients.

"*Insh'allah*," she said to the Arab patients, invoking God's mercy on their behalf. She would bend down to the little cots where children lay, cradle their faces in her hands and murmur, "*Shwaya, shwaya*, it's going to be okay."

When patients vomited she rubbed their backs and told them, "That's great! Keep going!" When patients cried in pain, she said, "You're a hero," or "You're so brave." Even to the sickest patients, patients we knew would likely die, Hannah said, "You're doing so well."

What a snow job, I thought. "Why do you say it's going to be okay for them?" I challenged her one day, "why give them false hope? Shouldn't we be helping them accept reality?"

Boy, do you have a lot to learn, said the look on Hannah's face. "There will be time for that. They need hope. Right now, hope is just as important as chemotherapy – maybe even more."

Patients loved her. "Hannah," a patient called to her. "I put out three hundred cc of urine. Is it enough?" "Don't worry," she answered, "I only put out two hundred cc myself." Another time, a patient who had been in remission for a year arrived in relapse. "Oh no, not you again!" Hannah said with the perfect lightness of touch to wring a sad smile from him as she pulled him to her in a big hug.

"Damn it," growled Dr. Ben Cassis whenever he heard that one of his patients had relapsed.

THE BLOOD DRAWING had to be completed by precisely ten o'clock in the morning. If I was running late because I had difficulty finding veins or was conversing with the patients too much, Aviva came over to help me finish up, and I soon found out why. All the doctors, nurses, secretaries, and lab technicians gathered in a cramped office a few doors away from the clinic for breakfast, and it was not to be missed. Breakfast required the team's full attendance and during that time, the patients seemed to understand that they would have to fend for themselves and each other. Patients might be in the middle of treatments or receiving a blood transfusion, and others throwing up, but at 10:00 a.m. sharp, the team disappeared.

Out of nowhere, a huge spread appeared, laid out by Jamilla, a young girl from the West Bank who was the hired helper. The table was laden with a pot of strong brewed coffee, plates of green olives, soft white cheese, slices of yellow cheese, piles of hot toast, platters of cucumbers, radishes, red peppers, and a salad composed of tomatoes and cucumbers chopped into tiny pieces. As if we didn't have any pressing work or sick patients a few steps away, we sat down to enjoy a luscious, leisurely meal.

I usually sat perched on the edge of the sink where I could listen in on their loud, heated discussions in Hebrew. I didn't feel confident enough with the language to be a part of it and weigh in on any of the controversial topics they raised. They all held strong opinions about everything. They spoke about new chemotherapy protocols, the wins or losses of the Tel Aviv soccer team, the rising price of tomatoes, and, of course, politics. (Sometimes the price of tomatoes was a political issue in itself.) They spoke about plans for the soon-to-be-opened bone marrow transplant unit, and about economic cutbacks to health care, and the unrest just starting to brew on the West Bank, called the *intifadah*.

Hannah had explained to me how our Arab patients came to us. "The hospital bus brings them in the morning from the *occupied territories*," she started off, allowing a few extra seconds for that contentious phrase to sink into my brain. "They receive treatments and then the bus returns them to their homes in Gaza or the West Bank."

Once, I looked out the window of the clinic and saw a circle of Bedouin mothers eating their mid-morning meal of grapes, pita bread, and sunflower seeds. They lifted their veils to spit out the seeds and sat laughing and talking while minding their children who played all around them. A little boy stopped to pee in the sand. I chuckled to myself when I thought about how inadequate was the lecture I'd received on "cross-cultural nursing," where the professor had suggested we inquire, "Did the patient wear ethnic costume or Western dress?"

Hannah lit up a cigarette. "They know their child is sick and can't get proper medical treatment in their villages, but they don't like to come to us." She shook her head sadly and took a deep drag on her cigarette. "Slowly, they are gaining confidence in us, but if their village is put under curfew or they're hassled at the border after a terrorist attack, all is lost. Once, we sent an ambulance in to pick up kids for chemo treatments. At first, the mothers were scared when the soldiers came to get their kids, but then they understood what they were doing and kissed them. Have you noticed how blood tests make them very nervous? They're scared we'll take too much and they don't like getting Jewish blood, but they are relieved we don't ask for a blood donation in return. All in all, they're grateful but would rather not be dependent on us. Maybe one day, we'll all realize that disease is the enemy, not one another."

Aviva saw the situation differently. One morning at breakfast, she spoke about an Israeli soldier who was killed in a terrorist attack on the northern border. One of his kidneys had been transplanted into a ten-year-old Arab boy in renal failure, and she wasn't pleased about that. "Don't you think we should take care of our own, first?" she asked me, fuming.

"We must put all personal feelings aside," said Dr. Ben Cassis, coming into the room and pouring himself a cup of coffee. He was a dark-skinned Moroccan Jew who dressed for work formally in a suit and tie that he removed the moment he walked out the door at the end of each day. He was brilliant, but stern and unapproachable. "What we do here is pure, untainted by politics. That's the beauty of medicine."

It was unlike him to speak about the beauty of anything and it stirred me to hear him say that. I began to take more of an interest in him, though he was married and had teenaged kids. But not for one moment was it lost on me, the similarity of his name with my old television love interest, Dr. Ben Casey.

"Have you heard? There's been another devaluation of the currency," said Aviva, changing to her other favourite subject, numbers and facts, checks and balances. "Yesterday one thousand shekels was worth one thousand shekels. Today, it's the same, but tomorrow, one thousand shekels will equal one shekel. It's not just shifting a decimal point. Soon, our money will be worthless."

"It's because of the Lebanon campaign. We can't continue bombing Beirut," said Ben Cassis wearily. He seemed weary not just of the endless war or the politics, or the economic woes of the country. He was weary of treating cancer patients and losing so many of them. He was weary of life itself. "And the West Bank and Gaza Strip, too. It's time to pull out of there altogether."

"Last month, I earned three hundred and twenty dollars," Aviva continued. "It makes more sense to go into overdraft than to forgo something, 'cause the price will surely double by next month."

"If we even make it to next month," said Ben Cassis.

"Oh, shut the hell up," said Hannah good-naturedly, and we all had a good laugh.

I decided to plunge into the conversation and tell them about the drastic cutbacks in health care also taking place in Canada. It was so severe, I said, that there were no jobs for nurses. It seemed like health care was in crisis everywhere, I went on, but no one was paying the least bit of attention to what I was saying because they were all doubled over, howling with laughter. Aviva explained the joke to me. "The word for economic cutbacks is *ketzitzot*, not *ketzitzim*. You said there were drastic 'meatballs,' not 'cutbacks' in health care spending!" I laughed too, but hoped they weren't going to bring up the other grammatical blooper I'd made the day I left Hannah a note asking her to order more blankets. By accidentally substituting one letter in the word, I'd ended up asking her to order more "happiness" instead.

Hannah and Dr. Ben Cassis were always the positive and negative charge, the mother and the father of the unit. But there were times that not even the fun and banter of those communal morning meals made Ben Cassis lighten up.

"Yuri, Yuri," he said about the patient who had relapsed. "Damn it," he said, pounding his fist on the tabletop. He closed his eyes. "Oh, Yuri," he said sadly to himself.

"He's a Russian tragedy," said Hannah, pointing at Ben Cassis with her cigarette. "Yosef, did you examine Khalid today? He's looking better. He's even got a smidgen of colour in his cheeks."

"It's leftover hemoglobin from the three units of blood he got last week. He's not producing his own. Soon, when the Bleomycin we gave him destroys his lungs, we'll be visiting him in the Intensive Care Unit. He'll have to be on a ventilator. I'm sure he'll appreciate us then."

"How about Geula? She's improving."

"Geula?" Ben Cassis repeated. "None of her four children is a bone marrow match, and I have that news to tell her today."

"But she has more energy," said Hannah. "She's in good spirits."

"Her diarrhea is lessening," I offered.

"So, she'll die without diarrhea, so what? We give them a drug for the leukemia, but it destroys their liver. Another drug damages their kidneys. They get mouth sores, skin rashes, ulcers, and pain. The only question is will they die from the disease or from the treatment we're giving them?"

"We have to believe in what we are doing," Hannah said, trying to lighten the tone. "I gave chemo to my neighbour's dog and he's cured of leukemia. I believe in our treatments. It's all we have."

Ben Cassis sighed heavily. "I don't believe in anything. I certainly don't believe Geula will make it. She looks worse every single day."

"You are an unbearable human being." Hannah squinted at him through her cigarette smoke.

"The only thing that might help Geula is a blessing from the Rabbi," he said sarcastically.

"Isn't it enough that you are a man of no faith? What do you care if she goes to the Rabbi for a blessing?"

"Ceremony and ritual are abracadabra nonsense, but the laws of God and the laws of Science are one and the same."

"The family is praying every day," Hannah said.

"So am I. So am I," he said with a nasty laugh.

"Yosef, you're impossible." Hannah stubbed out her cigarette. "Well, Geula may die, but she will be happier getting there if she prays along the way. Let me ask, do you believe in anything?"

"Yes," he said, "in science."

"Hannah, I need you," a patient called out.

"Turn off the toaster," she said to Jamilla, and to the rest of us, "let's get back to work."

I could feel myself becoming dangerously attracted to Dr. Ben Cassis, but at times, his detached, rational approach put me off, and sometimes put off his patients, too. Once, I was assisting him with an examination and when he finished, as I helped the patient up off the table, she asked him when she should come back to see him again.

"In two weeks," he answered curtly.

She looked scared. "What if I don't make it till then?"

"In that case, you won't have to come back." He closed the chart, stood up, and walked to the door. The patient and I looked at each other. She turned to Ben Cassis in reproach, but he was gone, on to the next case. But I think we both understood that he hadn't meant to be cruel, merely logical.

A FEW MONTHS AFTER I began working in the clinic, the new bone marrow transplant unit was almost ready to be opened and Shoshana Zamir, as the Nursing Director, called a meeting of the entire team to discuss its organization and management. "Hannah Shalev will be the head nurse and Aviva Shofet her assistant," Shoshana announced.

"No, no, no," interrupted Hannah. She had no patience for titles or accolades. Her dangling earrings tinkled as she shook her head. "Aviva and I will share the head nurse position."

"There can never be two captains of a ship," Dr. Ben Cassis said, "never two generals of an army. There has to be a Chief-of-Staff and a second-in-command."

Hannah was older, wiser, and more experienced, but Aviva was much more ambitious, taking night courses at the university toward her nursing degree to get ahead. When Shoshana chose Hannah, Aviva tried to hide her disappointment, but I felt relieved. Although Aviva was helpful to me, she was also bossy and critical and always finding fault.

Shoshana Zamir had asked me to prepare some information on the nursing care of bone marrow transplant patients so that I could assist the other nurses with our new educational needs.

"Ahh, our little *professor*," said Hannah, blowing away a puff of smoke, as if to clear the way for me to make my presentation. "Why are you studying all the time?" she often asked me. Sure enough, at that meeting, she joked, "Nursing theories? What good are they? All bluff and blah-blah." My scalp tingled as I blushed in embarrassment. "Forgive me, Tilda, but I have no pretensions about what it is to be a nurse. I have no use for academics and philosophers who have forgotten that if they want to call themselves nurses, they should take care of patients. Nurses must never forget that their work is with patients, wiping their noses or their asses or whatever needs to be wiped. That's what nursing is about!"

"What about talking with patients and listening to their concerns? Isn't that nursing, too?"

"Of course it is, but too much digging and probing can do more harm than good. Listen, Tilda, a nurse is someone who helps people feel better. End of story."

That was Hannah's nursing theory. Well, one thing was for sure, you didn't have to read between the lines to figure out where you stood with her.

ONE OF THE FIRST patients admitted to the new unit was a high-ranking army officer named Shaul Dayan. The treatment we had given him for his multiple myeloma was successful, but he still got infections and mouth sores. Even so, he looked virile and handsome. One morning, Ben Cassis told me he wanted to perform a bone marrow biopsy on Shaul and so I began to gather everything he would need for the procedure. I rushed around, setting up as quickly as possible, as I could hear him pacing impatiently outside the door. I had to keep running in and out to retrieve things I'd forgotten and when I came back in, Shaul said, "Listen, don't let old Ben Cassis put pressure on you. This is what you will need for the procedure." He made me a list: gauze, sterile drapes, a Jamshidi (a specialized instrument for performing this type of biopsy), a large syringe, and an assortment of glass slides and containers for the samples of his own bone marrow. "Relax," he told me, handing me the list, "you can do it." Ben Cassis performed the difficult procedure, which involved puncturing the hip bone with a large needle and extracting a sample of bone marrow. (Most patients screamed during that test, but Shaul smiled.) Assisting with that procedure always upset me because I imagined how excruciating the patient's pain must be and I knew how much depended on the results. Afterwards, Ben Cassis left the room abruptly, and I stayed behind to tidy up. Shaul saw that I was distraught and put his arm around my waist to comfort me. I couldn't help but fall in love with him, too. In Shaul's case, that was a particularly easy thing to do and I was not the only one. Rarely a day or night passed when there was not a beautiful woman at his bedside.

"I am his wife," said a woman.

"I am his girlfriend," said one on a separate occasion.

"I am his lover," said another.

"I am his Commanding Officer," said yet another.

"I am his wife," said a different one, and I didn't ask any questions.

"I am his mother," said an older woman, and I could see the resemblance.

Boldly, I asked him about them and he grinned. "They all cry over me but I tell them they are allowed only one to two teardrops per day. But sometimes they exceed their quota."

On occasion, Shaul told me a little bit about his work in Intelligence for the Israeli Defence Force. "The wars of the seventies exposed some serious weaknesses in our land intelligence systems," he explained. "Today's battlefield is more demanding, with more deadly weapons, especially during counter-engagements. The old-fashioned methods of obtaining information through agents and interrogators have low effectiveness, especially when we need immediate, accurate information for the precise identification of targets. Remember Iraq, in 1981?"

"Were you involved in that?" I asked, but he only smiled in answer. "I developed electro-optical devices for remote-piloted vehicles that display targets in real time."

"I see," I said, trying to.

Later that day, Ben Cassis showed me the results of Shaul's bone marrow biopsy. "He's at his nadir," he said grimly. "He is vulnerable to infection. We'll have to put him in protective, reverse isolation."

Now, we had to approach him in gowns, gloves, and masks. It wasn't the usual type of isolation procedure where we were protecting ourselves from infection. In this case, we were trying to protect the patient from organisms we might be harbouring. Over the top of my mask, I smiled at Shaul with my eyes and he smiled back with all of him. "Are you cold?" I asked. "Here's a blanket."

"Put that down. Sit with me." He patted the bed beside him. "Here."

What did he need from me? He had all his army buddies and all those wives, girlfriends, and lovers who lavished attention upon him. And if Aviva caught me sitting, doing nothing, she would think me lazy. "I'd better go," I said, inching toward the door.

"Don't leave." He held me with his eyes. "Don't avoid me."

I hadn't realized I was doing that. His face was thin and pale, but in his eyes I saw his vitality. Suddenly I realized what he did in the army. It was obvious. He was a spy. He could fool anybody he wasn't going to die.

"Sit down," he said, "and be with me."

"Of course." I sat next to him on his bed. "I'm here. I'm with you."

"Breathe," he said, and we sat quietly for a few minutes. He handed me a pair of earphones and he put on his and plugged both into his tape recorder. "Listen to this."

"It's magnificent," I said, still breathing for him.

"Of course it is." He grinned. "It's Bach's *Magnificat*." He lowered the volume. "Tilda, when two people listen to music together, it is an act more intimate than sex. Music is direct experience, the only one that two people can feel at the same time. Even during love making each person is inside their own orgasm, experiencing their private pleasure. Only music can be felt simultaneously."

I was loath to change the subject but I had to ask him something. "Shaul, are you afraid?"

He thought a moment. "Not of death," he said, "only of pain." He had started to suffer terrible bone pain and could no longer be as stoic as he had been for the biopsy. Once, his pain was so bad that I gave him a large injection of morphine very quickly. His eyes rolled back and he went limp. I was afraid I'd given too much, too fast. "Shaul," I shouted at him. "Are you there?"

"Don't worry, sweetheart," he answered with his eyes closed. "I feel fantastic. I love you."

IN THOSE DAYS, I had the ability to block everything out of my mind on my days off. I had some mental switch that allowed me to disconnect from any thoughts of my patients and their problems. I put it all out of my mind and escaped into fabulous adventures with the new friends I was making. We went camping in the desert, scuba diving in the Red Sea, had mud packs in the Dead Sea, went skinny-dipping in the Sea of Galilee, and went horseback riding through the Golan Heights. We threw parties and sang, drank, and danced all night. On many occasions, I went up to Jerusalem with them and we visited the holy sites there. Once, while standing in the *shuk*, the outdoor market where vendors had overflowing displays of vegetables, fruits, nuts, seeds, and spices, all bursting with colour and flavour (I never knew there were so many varieties of olives, dates, pecans, and pomegranates), I thought about my father and burst into tears. He would have loved that panoply and to have tasted each item, so I did, as many as I could, in his stead.

Every month, I called my mother and tried to have a conversation, but it was impossible to hear her and what I heard I could not understand. Just as my frustration was about to spill over into anger, Pearl came on at the right moment and helped me say goodbye and hang up.

THERE WERE FIVE single-patient rooms in the bone marrow transplant unit; two nurses worked on days and one nurse at night when it was usually quieter. Since I was the most junior, I ended up being assigned to more night shifts than the others. At first I was worried about working alone, but Hannah assured me I could call her at home if I had any questions and the doctors and nurses in the main ward, Barrack Thirty-six, were always available to help if needed.

One evening Ayelet, the day nurse, gave me her report as I came in to start my night shift. Shaul was now in remission and had gone home a few days ago. In his bed was Talia Bar-Lev, who was six days post–bone marrow transplant. She was doing well, except for persistent high fevers, which could indicate lingering infection, but tonight they had abated. Abdullah, a twelve-year-old boy from Gaza, was to be discharged the next day. His mother watched over him and nodded at me when I checked in on him. Yuri was there that night, too. He was to get a bone marrow transplant in a few days, but seemed relaxed, sitting up and watching TV when I peeked in on him. In the fourth bed was Samuel Abulafia with his wife sleeping in a chair beside his bed. He had been admitted that morning in pulmonary edema, a buildup of fluid in his lungs, but for now, he seemed comfortable and was breathing easily.

"Only four patients?" I looked at the fifth room. An empty bed might not stay that way.

"I haven't heard about anyone who needs it." Ayelet got up to leave. "I know it's a nurse's superstition, but I'll say it, anyway. It's been a slow day. I'm pretty sure you'll have a quiet night."

After I got everyone settled for bed, I did a final check. The patients were comfortable and stable. Talia had been started on a new medication and her fever was now down. Yuri's TV was on softly, but I knew he'd leave it on all night. He had told me once how he dreaded falling asleep, afraid he might not wake up. I stood in the doorway, chatting with him for a few moments and told him I was close by if he needed anything. Then I lowered the lights in the hall and at the nurses' station. Abdullah's mother had spread out a mat on the floor and was reciting her night prayers outside her son's room. When she finished she came and stood observing me over the counter, smiling at me from behind her black veil. Each time I caught her watching me, she giggled and looked away. I was writing in my journal, where I recorded my private thoughts every day. I felt her watching my pen move across the page. She opened a picnic basket and offered me a banana. It was two in the morning. The long night stretched ahead of us. We both yawned at the same moment. I handed her a stack of lab reports and a rubber stamp, and she was pleased to help me while I prepared medications for the morning. Then she sat down on a chair beside me. There we were, the two of us, unable to speak to one another, but understanding each other perfectly. Soon we fell asleep, leaning heavily into each other, our heads resting on the tabletop. A sharp knock at the back door startled me awake. It was 3:00 a.m. Geula's husband stood on the doorstep with his wife in his arms.

"She's vomiting blood," he cried. I saw the trail behind him. "Bring her in," I said. "Put her in the bed." I pointed to the empty room.

Although he hadn't predicted this crisis would happen so soon, Ben Cassis had spoken about this very possibility yesterday on rounds. Geula had received a bone marrow transplant from an unknown donor. The match was good, but not perfect, and he'd seen ominous signs of "graft versus host" syndrome. It is the opposite of what occurs in organ transplants where the person, the "host," may reject the organ, the "graft." In GVH, the transplanted bone marrow is seen as a foreign body and is rejected by the recipient.

Luckily, Ben Cassis had left explicit orders in the case of this eventuality and I got to work. I quickly inserted a naso-gastric tube down her nose and into her stomach to drain the blood. Then I started an IV for fluids, another for antibiotics and steroids, and another for blood and platelet transfusions. I hung the first unit of blood. As I waited until the tubing blushed, pinked up, became crimson, and then deepened to scarlet, I searched Geula's face for signs of life being revived within her. I had seen blood have fast, almost magical effects, but Geula lay there, limp and pale, barely conscious. Her four daughters gathered around her bed, chanting prayers and a song with a haunting melody:

   The entire world is only a narrow bridge
   The main thing – the main thing – is never to be afraid.

The youngest daughter, Sarah, who was only nine years old, nestled into the curve of her mother's bent legs. The older girls dabbed at her forehead and lips with water that had been blessed by the Chief Rabbi of Israel. I recalled Geula's last admission, just after her bone marrow transplant and how the family had moved into the same room she was in now. In no time it became full of puzzle books, homework notes and textbooks, and a row of their sandals lined up along the wall by the door. I had a feeling that during this admission there would be no time to set up camp as before.

I recalled meeting Geula and her family in the out-patient clinic. I had asked Tikva, the eldest daughter, a question that opened the floodgates: "Tell me about your mother before she got sick."

"My mother is a successful business woman. She owns a textile factory. She knew from the start how serious her situation was, yet she always said she would beat this thing. Even after each chemo treatment she got up and went to work. We aren't close, but she's my mother, you know?"

I nodded. *Yes, I knew about mothers.*

Tikva usually spoke for the family and approached me now. "Nurse Teelda, please don't give my mom any sedation. We want her to be with us the whole time, even if tonight is the end."

"Even if she is in pain?" I asked.

"Well, maybe then," she conceded, "but we want her to know we are with her."

This was a matter for a longer discussion, but I had to check on Abdullah and Talia. Both were sleeping quietly. Suddenly, I heard Samuel start coughing violently. I ran to him and found him struggling to sit up in bed, spitting frothy blood into a linen hand-kerchief. He gasped for air. I raised the head of his bed, gave him an oxygen mask, and administered Lasix that had been ordered for him if this happened. It would increase his urine output and thereby reduce the excess fluid load on his heart and lungs.

"I'm sorry it's taking so long," he whispered.

What, to die? He's sorry it's taking so long?

"I'm ready," he said, gasping for air. "It's my time."

I knew he had decided on no more treatment, but I had to make him more comfortable. I gave him a small injection of morphine and stood beside him waiting. Would the sparrows still come to him in the morning if he were too weak to sing for them, I won-dered? That very morning, they had heard his calls and had flown right into his room in the barrack. His wife held his hand and I smoothed his brow and watched his breathing start to ease. *Blessed morphine*, I thought.

"Am I in heaven?" Samuel asked.

Why not let him think so, if that would comfort him? I guess I had learned a thing or two from Hannah by then. I nodded yes. Was it lying? If so, I didn't care. I bent down and kissed his dear fore-head. I had never done something that intimate to a patient before.

I stood there and began to weep, for him, for Shaul, and for all of the patients that we'd lost and were going to lose.

"Nurse Teelda?" Tikva stood at the door. "Come now, please! Mom needs you."

I hurried out of Samuel's room and rushed past Yuri's room where the TV was still on. It was 3:30 a.m. and despite himself, he'd fallen asleep, the remote control still in his hand. Abdullah's mother watched me. I felt she wanted to help me but didn't know what to do, so she stayed by her son's side as if to indicate that she would tend to him if he needed anything and thus lighten my load by at least one patient. For the rest of that night, as I rushed from patient to patient, I felt the weight of each decision I made, of each

action I took or did not take. Each one held a practical implication, but also a huge moral freight, too. If I ran to hang another
unit of blood for Geula, I might not get to Samuel in time to suction
him and he would suffer and be afraid. If I stopped to readjust
Samuel's oxygen mask and comfort his wife, Geula's naso-gastric
tube might clot off. Talia was sleeping peacefully, but she was due
for medications and they would have to be given late. I kept
running as fast as I could in all directions, doing as much as I could.

Tikva was getting frantic. "When will Dr. Ben Cassis be here?"
she asked.

"In the morning," I said. It was almost 5:00. I imagined him in
bed lying beside his wife.

"How could God do this to us?" the daughters cried, standing around their mother's bed. The husband sat in a chair,
sobbing. Geula's breathing was raspy and heavy. They understood that her kidneys had stopped working. They saw the pools
of blood all around her. "Do something!" Tikva shouted at me.
"Do something!"

It was 6:00 a.m. In an hour everyone would be there. "The
doctor is on his way," I said to them. I looked out the window,
scanning the horizon for the sun. The night sky was giving way to
a violet sky with streaks of orange that promised that day would
come. I looked at the mess I'd made. Empty vials and used syringes
were strewn all over the counter. I had thrown a drained bag of
blood at a garbage can and missed and I watched the last few drops
drip onto the floor.

"You should have called us," they all said when they arrived, but
I could tell I had won their respect for having toughed out the night
on my own. Aviva got straight to work tidying up, shaking her head
at the disorder. Ben Cassis sat down and started grilling me about
each patient. "What did you do then?" he asked. "Next? . . . What
then?" He seemed satisfied with each answer I gave, but kept on
going. Hannah went into the tiny on-call room, off of the nurses'
station and left the door open so that she could see and hear everything. She wanted to intervene and tell him to lighten up, but didn't
dare interrupt. Jamilla arrived with her friend Fredja and they were

chattering and laughing as they started up their little *finjan* on the stove to brew Turkish coffee and then began the morning *sponja*. Aviva wiped off the countertops. "Whose medication is this?" she asked. She held up a syringe filled with clear yellow fluid. I stared at it in her hand.

"How did Talia deal with the high dose of Amphotericin?" Dr. Ben Cassis continued his interrogation. "Did she have a reaction this time? Any chills or rigours? What's her temperature?"

"A reaction?" I asked slowly, stalling, thinking it through.

"I hope you gave it slowly, with lots of fluid. Did you do that?"

No, I hadn't given it at all. I had prepared it and drawn it out of the vial, but I hadn't given it to Talia. I gulped for air, but my throat closed up tight. "I forgot to give it," I squeaked. Aviva ran off to tend to Geula as I stood stock-still, quaking in terror, staring at that syringe on the counter.

"What? How could you be so stupid?" Ben Cassis pounded his fist on the tabletop. "Damn it!" he shouted. Hannah jumped up. I thought he might hit me, but words were his blows. "You could have killed her," he screamed at me, switching to English, as if its foreignness might help him restrain himself from murdering me. Maybe he did it to even the playing field, otherwise it would be like crushing a bug. He was a powerful, intimidating man, but he was not a bully.

"I know, I know," I cried.

"Surely you realize that a patient as immuno-compromised and vulnerable as Talia could quickly become septic!" he raged at me. "She could die from a fungal infection!"

I stood there taking it. I deserved it. It was part of my punishment.

"This is a matter of life and death here! Don't you realize that?" I nodded and looked down at my blood-splattered running shoes. "If Talia dies, it is because of your carelessness."

"That's enough." Hannah stood in between us. "Go home," she whispered to me. "Talia will live or die regardless of one missed dose." I couldn't move. Hannah took my face in her hands. "Go home, sweetie. You need sleep. See you tonight." She pushed me toward the door. Dizzy and exhausted, I stumbled out and onto the dirt road at the back of Barrack Thirty-six Alef. As I began to make my way home, the wailing began. Geula's daughters' grief shook the old building.

I reviewed the night. I must have reasoned that Talia, the youngest and the most curable, could likely withstand more temporary neglect than the others. Although the others had less chance of survival, I felt certain Talia would make it through the night. And even though we were not actively treating Samuel any more, I had to ensure he was comfortable and didn't suffer. Geula's fierce daughters intimidated me and I was afraid they would blame me if she died during the night, while I was alone on duty. So, even though Geula had been closest to death, I had worked the hardest on her. My thought process was flawed because it was motivated by fear.

I made it home and didn't even bother to shower before flopping onto my bed, still in my uniform. I tried to sleep. The phone rang and I jumped up. As I flew to it, I felt certain it was Ben Cassis calling to tell me that Talia had died. I answered the call and instead took a message for my roommate to call her mother. Finally, I fell asleep and when I woke up it was ten o'clock that night, barely time to rush back to work by eleven o'clock for another night shift.

That night new patients were in Samuel's and Geula's beds, now freshly washed and made up, completely innocent of the suffering they had recently contained. Yuri was watching the TV show *Top of the Pops*, the weekly hit parade of tunes, and waved to me as I walked past. Abdullah had been discharged home that morning. Only his mother and I knew what had gone on that night.

For months after that night, I avoided Ben Cassis. Of course, I worked with him and saw him every day, but I never made eye contact with him. I felt cowed in his presence and kept a low profile. I started getting headaches before going in to work and I checked and double-checked myself even more than ever. How could he ever trust me again? I asked Hannah for some time off, but she told me she didn't have anyone to cover my shifts.

A FEW MONTHS LATER, on another night shift, I had an opportunity to make peace with Ben Cassis. I took over from the day nurse and she gave me report about Dawud, a twenty-two-year-old man from Gaza, recently diagnosed with leukemia. He was coughing up blood and his blood pressure was low. Shortly after she left, I took my own reading and could barely detect it. His pulse was weak and thready. He was cool and clammy. I opened up his IV and let fluid pour in and called Ben Cassis at home and reported my findings.

"He's gone into septic shock," he said to me. "Damn it," he said to himself. He began to outline exactly what he wanted me to do: give lots of fluid, plus two units of packed red blood cells, ten units of platelets, start him on a different, stronger antibiotic and a drug I wasn't familiar with called Dopamine. "What's that?" I had to ask him because there was no time to look it up as I was taught to always do. "Dopamine is a powerful drug that will constrict the vasculature," he explained, "and it will raise the blood pressure." I hung up the phone and got to work.

"Ya! Allah!" cried his young wife along with his mother and sisters, who gathered around his bed. "Ya! Allah!" they wailed and threw themselves upon his body. They had turned his bed around to face Mecca, in case he should die before the morning. As I hung the first unit of blood, I looked up to see Dr. Ben Cassis walking in the door. For the rest of that night we worked side by side. I gave the antibiotics and assisted him as he inserted a central line into the patient's subclavian vein through which I could run the Dopamine faster and more safely. I took care of the other patients while he stayed with Dawud. At dawn, we took a break and sat down at the nurses' station. I thought about Aviva and what she'd say when she arrived in the morning. She would look at the mess and exclaim, "You made all this effort for a guy who might go on to bomb us?"

He looked at me and, as if reading my mind, said, "We must never hesitate." He raked his fingers through his dark hair. "The Arabs hate us and don't want us in the West Bank or the Gaza Strip. I dare say they don't want us in Tel Aviv or Haifa, either. The bottom line is that they don't want us here at all. However, we must have no hesitation whatsoever about what we do as doctors and nurses."

I got up to make us coffee and when I returned I saw to my utter embarrassment that he was reading my journal that I had accidentally left out on the desk at the nurses' station. Because he had opened it from right to left as he would a Hebrew book, he wasn't reading about my wild adventures and fantasies (many involving him) but rather from the few pages at the back where I kept a running list of the patients who had died, along with a few details to always remind me of each one.

"Why do you do this?" he asked sadly. To him it was a list of his failures.

"It's how I remember them," I explained. He looked at me. He stood up and drew me into his arms. I could feel his breath on my hair. "Oh, Teelda," he said in that ice cream way they all had of saying my name. Then he kissed me. The thought of war and enemies so close by was such a turn-on. (Funny how peace and reconciliation doesn't have the same effect.) I wanted to stay in his arms as long as possible, but within seconds, I felt the kiss melting away and the hug petering out.

I HAD BEEN in Israel almost a year to the day when I got home from work one evening to find a message on the answering machine from Pearl: "Your mother is sick, man. She had a stroke and is in the hospital, but she is okay. Good enough. God is love."

It was spring and once again the sweet smell of the orange blossoms in the groves near the hospital filled the air. The hills in the cow pasture were covered in wildflowers. Just as everything was coming into bloom, I had to tear myself away from it all, and return to my dreary responsibilities back home. As I packed up to go, I thought back over the year. Talia was completely cured and in her first year of law school. Abdullah was in remission. Yuri was feeling great and came to visit us with his girlfriend to tell us they were engaged. Dawud made it through that difficult night, but died a few months later. Shaul was at home dealing with terrible bone pain. I didn't inquire about any of the others. I was leaving.

Ben Cassis said goodbye. "You are a fine young woman and an excellent nurse. I'm glad we didn't ruin you. We wish you well." But he must have known what I felt for him because he tenderly touched my cheek as tears dripped down my face. He bent down to speak softly to me. "We're friends," he said, "and friendship is more important than love. Remember that."

Aviva and Hannah hugged me and then I got into a taxi and headed for the airport.

5

HARDER, FASTER

Straight from the airport, I took a taxi to my mother in the hospital. She lay in a bed, the side rails up around her, unmoving and unresponsive. I don't think she saw me, much less recognized me.

"She's beeyootiful." Pearl fluffed her hair with a brush. "Getting better every day."

My mother was now bedridden and paralyzed. She could no longer eat and had to be fed through a tube. Now that she required around-the-clock nursing care, the hospital had become her home, but Pearl continued to visit her. My mother spoke very little, but as I got up to leave, I heard her mutter, "I wish I had a daughter like her."

My mother's home had been sold, so that night I stayed at my friend Joy's house. Her mother, Bunny, took one look at me and seemed to understand how bad things were.

"Just take it one day at a time," she said, soothingly.

I couldn't bring myself to tell her that I was so low I was going minute by minute.

The next day I went back to my mother and this time she was
sitting up in bed and more alert, but was very agitated. "You and
your friends are going to jail," she said when she saw me.

"See, her head stay up when you're here, girl," Pearl exclaimed.
"For you!"

"She's not making any sense."

"But when she open her mouth to sing, the voice is there, right
there!" Pearl slapped the back of one hand into the palm of the
other. "You can't add to it and you can't take away from it."

"Don't close that on me!" my mother cried out.

"Close what, my dear?" Pearl bent down and put her arm
around her and leaned her dark head close to my mother's colour-
less lips. "What is it, love?"

I fled from them both and descended into the subway and rode
the train for hours. Those subway tunnels became my sub-
terranean hideout. There wasn't much I could do for my mother
any more and I knew I had to start looking for a job, but I couldn't
face it right away. I needed to be alone. So, between short visits to
my mother in the hospital, I rode the subway thinking things over.
I tried to block out my grief over my family situation and the
yearning I felt for the exciting life I'd left behind in Israel. I stayed
underground, riding for hours, thinking things over. Sometimes I
just rode, my mind completely empty. I would doze off for a few
hours here and there, and manage to get enough sleep that I could
walk all night through the city streets.

"SURE, YOU COULD STAY HERE, I guess . . ." my brother Stephen
said slowly when I showed up one evening on the doorstep of his
new condo in my subway clothes and tangled hair. Kindness had
never been his strong suit but it was a failing he was trying to
correct. "When did you get back from Israel?"

"A few weeks ago. I've sort of lost track of time." As I followed
after him, I caught an appalling glimpse of a scruffy, unwashed
hobo person in the hallway mirror.

"Well, come on in." If he was reluctant to let my unsightly,
unwashed self into his home, he was charitable enough not to

show it. He settled into a black leather chair and chomped on a cigar. "I have to tell you, Til, you're looking rather unkempt. You've got to pull yourself together." He continued on in this new, amiable vein. "Well, you're welcome to stay as long as you like. At least until you get your act together." He looked me over. "How long do you think that might take?"

I stayed overnight. As I slept, the sections of his leather couch would slip apart and I had to keep getting up to shove them back together. I tried to hold myself still so they wouldn't separate, but by the morning I was balancing on the middle section, my legs off one end, my head suspended off the other end, like a damsel on a magician's levitation table. By then, Stephen had left for work. I wrote him a thank-you note, left it on the dining room table, and went back underground. It was easier to live like a rat, wander the streets, sleep under bridges or in bushes, eat garbage, ride the subway all day, and not think about anything, rather than face my life.

Of course, I was still a nurse, but I had sunk into such a pit of depression and self-pity that the prospect of taking care of others, of assuming responsibilities as I had done in Israel, and hardest of all – having to be empathetic to other people's problems – seemed too much for me. For a while, I couldn't imagine I'd ever be able to be a nurse again. But after a few more miserable weeks of living a vagabond life and a scary glimpse of where I was about to end up, I managed to pull myself together and make myself passably presentable to apply for work. I signed on with a nursing agency on a freelance basis and started off with private duty assignments, caring for people in their homes after an illness or surgery such as a hip or knee replacement. The clients were wealthy and had high expectations of tip-top "customer service" from their nurses. One woman summoned me by ringing a silver bell! It made me feel like one of her little dogs. In fact, in addition to nursing care, I was also expected to run errands, do her shopping, and walk those dogs for her, but at least they were a lot friendlier than she was.

On another assignment in the home of a man recovering from a stroke, I had no sooner arrived when his wife imperiously told me to "rearrange his luggage." It seemed she wanted me to reposition his testicles while he was sitting in the wheelchair. I was uncomfortable with this instant familiarity, this required intimacy, just because I was a nurse. When the wife was out of earshot, and I was doing as she asked, the husband gave me a lurid grin. "Harder, faster," he whispered. All day he kept trying to touch my breasts and at one point, actually grabbed at my crotch. I stayed till the end of the shift, but told the agency I would not go back there, without explaining why. I felt I should have been able to put a stop to him myself. After all, I had defied Yaffa and refused to wear a cap. I had been in charge of the bone marrow transplant unit. But now, I was reduced to this – servant, dog-walker, baby-sitter, and now sex object!

As bad as it was, it was also a productive period in its own way. It helped me get back on my feet and after a few weeks I had enough cash to put down first and last months' rent on an apartment. I found a tiny bachelorette in a rough, down-and-out neighbour-hood but it was the start of a home for myself.

After a few months of those relatively cushy assignments, I was feeling stronger and ready to request a more demanding placement in a hospital. I got there early, feeling nervous as I walked slowly to the medical-surgical floor of a large downtown hospital where I'd been assigned, trying to steel myself for what might be thrown at me. There was always a sense of the unpredictable and that I might be expected to deal with more than I could handle.

That day I had eight patients who needed a great deal of nursing care. It seemed overwhelming but luckily, Scott, a Registered Practical Nurse, was working with me. Whatever superior attitude or reservation I might have had about working together with an RPN, a nurse with a more rudimentary nursing training than I, van-ished in minutes when I saw how skilled and professional he was. Not only was Scott an excellent nurse but his constant patter of jokes kept my flagging spirits buoyed.

"C'mon, girlfriend, let's go." He pushed a linen cart alongside us. "Most of our patients are NFW, and we have a few who are FVB." I shot him a questioning glance and he explained: "'Not Feeling Well and Feeling Very Bad.' But no sweat, most are walkie talkies."

"Come again?"

"Up and about, walking and talking. Don't worry. You'll get used to me."

A woman with curly grey hair wearing a bright blue terrycloth robe approached us. "My bed hasn't been changed in three days." Scott gathered up fresh sheets and we followed her into her room. "The service here is terrible," she said, supervising our work. "I'm going to transfer to another hospital."

We moved on to the next room where a patient was lying in a huge bed, under loads of covers. She was morbidly obese and bloated, too, from a buildup of fluid due to liver failure. She was so swollen it was difficult for her to get up or even move her body. She was scheduled for a procedure to insert a temporary shunt to drain the excess fluid from her body, but it was a stopgap measure at best. Only a new liver would save her life.

"When can I book my transplant?" she asked me.

"It doesn't quite work like that," I said but didn't have the time to explain the complex process.[*] Scott and I helped her to get up and out of bed and wash herself and then he took her vital signs and I gave her her medications. I looked at my watch and spurred myself to move faster. We still had six more patients to see. *A good nurse is a fast nurse. A fast nurse is a good nurse. Work harder, faster,* I told myself.

There were so many patients to see and problems to attend to. I spent entire shifts running to and fro, popping in and out of patients' rooms. I'd get one patient out of bed, run to give a medication, then have to dash off to answer a call bell. Wherever I was, I always felt like I was supposed to be somewhere else, dealing with something even more urgent. Everywhere I turned there was someone in distress. Patients were crying out or short of breath. They were sad or angry, wandering off or calling out, and many were confused, demented, and even hostile. There was no point lingering in a patient's room or delving too much into anyone's problems, as that would only create more information to chart and

---

[*] Here's a simplified version: One has to be sick enough to require a liver transplant, but not too sick that it would be overly risky. Of course, there has to be an organ donor, too.

make me get too far behind in my work. The work seemed never-ending, but I did see other nurses handling it quite capably. Some even stopped to chat with patients or share a laugh, but I never felt organized enough or fast and efficient enough to take the time. But the main reason was that I knew my ability to listen and be empathetic was limited by my preoccupation with my own problems. How far I felt from being that "therapeutic presence" the professors had extolled, or from being a member of a dynamic team like I had been in Israel. Exhausted and miserable, I kept at it. I got by and, thankfully, so did my patients.

WORKING FOR A NURSING AGENCY, I never knew where I would be sent and I rarely returned to the same floor two shifts in a row. The agency would call me early in the morning or late at night to inform me where my next gig would be. After a few months, I had worked in so many different hospitals that it was becoming a blur of patients and their crises and all I was left with was my constant and nagging feeling of inadequacy. One morning, at five o'clock, the supervisor called to say they were sending me to an ICU. I quickly reminded them I didn't have the qualifications to care for critically ill patients. I had to refuse that assignment, but it got me thinking about what it might be like to work in an ICU. Like the operating room or the emergency department, the ICU was a specialized area where many nurses aspired to work. Perhaps it was time to look for a permanent job and become part of a real team?

There was a patient I cared for during that time who I will never forget. My only regret is that I never returned to find out what happened to him. I choose to believe that he got better and is out there somewhere, crooning "Blue Suede Shoes." Tom Buckley was a spry seventy-year-old, originally from Newfoundland, who had worked as an Elvis impersonator for parties and events. He'd even won contests, boasted his girlfriend, Iris, especially when he sang "Love Me Tender." He was a jolly, stocky man who was always smiling. Iris was constantly at his side, dolled up in gaudy costume jewellery, thick pancake make-up, and a huge coral lipstick smile. She called him "Buddy," and so did we, the nurses. He was scheduled for a coronary artery bypass, but a CT scan* revealed that he also had a large aortic aneurysm, a potentially lethal condition. For days, the cardiovascular and the thoracic surgeons discussed the prospect of the complicated surgery he required as each staked out a claim to their portion of the patient's inner organs.

I wanted to follow up with Buddy so I asked the agency to send me back to that ward the next day. I wanted to go to him first, but I had to see a few other patients beforehand. I knew immediately that it wasn't going to be easy to establish any kind of "therapeutic relationship" with my first patient. She took one look at me and slammed down the phone on whomever she'd been talking to. "Fuck you, Maggie!" she yelled, pointing a long, manicured finger at me. Gospel music played loudly from a radio on her bedside table.

In these situations, we had been taught to say, "You seem angry. Do you want to talk about what's bothering you?" but I had no desire to step into the maelstrom of her anger. I kept it short and sweet. "How are you feeling this morning, Miss Wilson?"

"How the hell do you think I am? And I'm not taking any of those fuckin' pills of yours."

We will lift up to the Lord. Sing in Jesus' name. She began to hum along and snap her fingers, more to block out my presence and ignore me, I felt, than in worship. "I'm Tilda. I'm your nurse and I'm here to give you your antibiotics," I said, nodding at her IV.

"You can call me L'il Roxy. That's my stage name. Now you get the fuck out of here, Maggie, unless you got any painkillers on you! I told you never to come back. Oh, you can tidy up this shithole before you leave."

"You must be confusing me with someone else. Who is Maggie?"

She didn't answer. "And don't you touch my catheter or steal my pee. I have to measure what goes in and what comes out."

The nurse-client relationship is based on trust, I recalled reading somewhere. *Displacement of anger is a defence mechanism they'd taught us in Introduction to Psychology. Come back*

---

* Stands for Computerized Tomography (in full, Computerized Axial Tomography, or CAT). It's a scan that has the capacity to look deeply into the body.

later and take her vital signs, I told myself. *Let another nurse change her dressing. Move on.*

There were six more patients to get to before I could reward myself with a visit to Buddy and Iris. I gathered the supplies I would need to do a large dressing change, and as I was about to enter the room, another nurse saw me. "Brace yourself for that one," she advised, not explaining further.

I opened the door and immediately smelled something bad. The patient was a young woman who had undergone radical surgery for breast cancer, and I introduced myself to her.

Suppurating, I told myself, *is the fancy way to say 'full of pus.'* *Suppurating, suppurating*, I thought over and over like a mantra, as I peeled back thick layers of gauze that covered a huge, gaping, ragged incision that looked like it had been made with a hatchet. Her wound had become horribly infected and the sweetish, putrid smell was overwhelming. Rivulets of sticky green and yellow pus dripped down onto her gown and onto the bed. I tried to hide my revulsion. I swallowed hard and looked away.

"The other nurses wear a mask," the patient said. "In fact, they wear two masks and dab a few drops of mouthwash in between the layers. They say it helps. You'll know for next time."

Suddenly, I gagged. I ran out of the room and made it to a garbage can and vomited. When I came back I saw the patient had managed to dispose of the dirty bandages and had cleaned her wound and covered it with clean sterile gauze by herself. "I'm so sorry," I said.

Finally, I went to Buddy. "How are you feeling today?"

"Better than dead! You're the one who looks stressed." He settled back into his pillows. "Hey, Miss Tilda, have you seen my rash?"

"Rash?" I searched my notes. "Where do you have a rash?"

"On my skin. That's the best place for a rash!"

Iris and I exchanged exasperated looks. "That's bad, Buddy. Really bad," she said.

"What's for lunch, dearie?" he chirped when I brought him his tray. He lifted the cover and made a face. "Back home, at midday, I always have two poached eggs, side by each." He turned to Iris.

"You know what we'll do, dearie? We'll take Tilda home with us, screech her in, and make her kiss the codfish.* Then we'll prepare her a Jiggs' dinner."

"What's that?" I sat down on a chair beside his bed, wishing I could stay there all day.

"Salt beef, carrots, turnips, potatoes, sometimes an old rubber boot."

"Buddy puts a bit of salt beef in, on Sunday, for sure. Moose, if we can get it."

"Horse, if we can't. And guests. See, if we runs out of horse, then we use the guests!"

"Don't mind Buddy." Iris shook her head.

"Are you okay, Buddy?" I asked when he suddenly winced. "Are you having pain?" He rubbed his back and his chest. "Oh, it's pain, all right," he said. "It's good pain. Real good pain."

"The pain is good?"

"Yes, it's shocking good pain."

I ran to get him a painkiller and even before I gave it, he grinned at me. "Works like a charm," he said. "You're an angel."

Later that day, I had no choice but to face Miss Wilson, again, the woman who called me Maggie. She wasn't in her room when I went in to restart her IV, which had become displaced from her vein. I was just about to leave when I noticed a stack of loose sheets of paper on her bedside table. I HATE MY NURSE, she'd written in big letters. On another piece, in capital letters, FAT WHITE ASS and THERE'S A NURSE IN THIS HOSPITAL THAT I HATE. On another sheet, she'd written, SHE HAS IT IN FOR ME. SHE'S TRYING TO KILL ME. As I left her room, I twisted around to take a look at myself. *Was it really that fat?*

I came back later and tried to win her over. "How about a back rub?" I offered, but she said I was too rough. "Get me a Coke. I'm the captain and you're the skipper. Don't forget that."

---

* A screech-in is a Newfoundland hospitality *rite de passage* to initiate newcomers to the province, which involves dipping a foot in the ocean and literally kissing a cod.

"I have to restart your IV. It's gone interstitial, which means it's not in the vein properly." I could hear the anger mounting in my voice.

"You're talking too loudly. I'm not deaf." She glared at me. "I want another nurse to do it."

Why does she hate me? It was so unfair and unfounded! Did she hate me because I'm white? It was prejudice! She didn't give me a chance. Later, I went back to try again. *Surely, we could work out our differences, whatever they were?* I waited a few moments in her room. When she emerged from the bathroom, she came toward me carrying a measuring cup of urine she had drained from her catheter. I saw what she was about to do. "Don't even think about it," I warned her. "Don't you dare!"

"Oh, I dare!" she laughed, and flung the urine at me. I jumped out of the way just in time to have it splash on my pants and shoes. "That's for reading my private notes, you bitch."

Worse than urine, I was covered in humiliation. I wanted to flee to the locker room to shower and change my uniform but just then I heard an announcement that stopped me in my tracks. "Code Blue, Code Blue." *A cardiac arrest right here on this floor!* I knew who it was. Buddy's aneurysm must have blown or else he had gone into cardiac arrest. I ran into his room, following after the doctor and the respiratory therapist. A nurse had already gotten there and was on his bed doing chest compressions. Another nurse was pushing an IV medication right into Buddy's vein and another was setting up the defibrillator to shock his heart. I stepped back to let the more experienced nurses take over and ran to get them things they needed. The arrest continued on and I went out to the hall where Iris was waiting. She tugged at my sleeve. "What's happening?"

"They're working on him. They will try to resuscitate him and then will probably take him straight to the operating room."

"Thank God. Does that mean he's getting better?"

I put my arm around her in answer.

As I was leaving to go home that evening, the nurse who had given me the heads-up about that nasty wound called out to me. "Hey, you okay?" she asked.

"Fine," I said, hurrying off. "No problem," I called back.

Riding home on the subway, I found a seat by myself and let the tears flow. Yes, I was sad about Buddy, but I was crying about my father, my mother, my family, and myself. I had my own problems. Why did the patients always get all the sympathy?

BECAUSE I WORKED FREELANCE, for an agency, I was never in one hospital long enough to learn how things worked. Nights were particularly difficult as I had to figure things out for myself, such as when to call the doctor at home and when not to. Late one evening, I needed a laxative for one of my patients and I decided to page the doctor. She didn't answer and after an hour, I paged again. Finally, she called back. "You're calling me now for that? You couldn't think of it earlier? I hate to think what you'd do in a Code Blue."

"Okay, I'll just chart 'MD notified.'"

"Oh, how you nurses love that phrase so you can pass the buck! Calling me about some trivial thing you could have figured out for yourself or planned for ahead of time."

She was right. It *was* one of the oldest tricks in the book. Fobbing off my responsibility instead of merely speaking up for what my patient needed. But in most hospitals, a nurse couldn't even administer a laxative or a single Tylenol without a doctor's order. I went to my patient, but by then he was sound asleep and I wasn't about to wake him to give him milk of magnesia. There were so many situations like that, where nurses' hands were tied. But most times, the stakes were a great deal higher than a laxative. Once, near the end of my shift with a mountain of charting still to complete, a call bell rang. It wasn't one of my patients, so I let it ring. *Let someone else go*, I thought. But it kept ringing. I got up and went to answer it.

A man stood beside his bed, clutching his chest, his face crunched in agony. "Oh, I've never had such terrible pain," he groaned. I placed an oxygen mask over his face and called for help.

"I'll get you a painkiller." I eased him down onto the bed.

"Don't leave me." He clutched at my arm. "I'm dying. Get my wife."

I felt his pulse. It was rapid and strong. "I'll be right back," I said and ran for the electrocardiogram machine. I pushed it straight out ahead of me like a grocery cart and I was off on a madcap shopping spree. Running past the nurses' station, I called out for someone to bring morphine and an aspirin because I thought he might be having an acute coronary event – a heart attack.

"The doctor hasn't ordered it," the nurse in charge said, looking up over her glasses at me. "He's in emerge right now, seeing a patient. Wait till he gets here."

But if I waited, it might be too late. I was not authorized to give a medication that wasn't ordered, nor administer oxygen without a doctor's order, or even perform an ECG without an order, but this was an emergency and I went ahead and did all of those things.

Later, when the doctor finally arrived and the patient was feeling much better, he was furious. "I didn't order this ECG," he yelled at me and ripped it up. "Who do you think you are? If I report you, you'll lose your licence."

It turned out the patient had suffered a mild heart attack as I had suspected, but it was hardly reason to feel vindicated. It was a serious setback for the patient, but what seemed to concern the doctor much more was a nurse threatening his authority. It was an old, unspoken, unwritten "doctor-nurse game" you had to play and the rules stipulated that even if you, the nurse, knew something, you weren't supposed to let on. Diplomacy and tact were needed. Suggestions or hints were okay, but taking action and making decisions was far too bold. Even the nurse in charge backed up the doctor. "You are going to get yourself in trouble," she warned, but did concede, "You may actually have saved that guy's life. Maybe you really want to be a doctor?"

"No, I want to be a nurse," I mumbled. But I did want to be able to use my knowledge, skills, and judgment. I hated knowing what to do and being unable to do it; seeing things, but being unable to take action. The worst was feeling invisible and unheard.

WORKING FOR THAT AGENCY, I really got around. I worked in medical wards such as Neurology, Nephrology, or Cardiology, where patients had chronic problems such as diabetes, asthma, congestive heart failure, kidney problems, and in many cases a few, or all, of the above. Those wards were usually separate from other specialties like Orthopedics, General Surgery, or Gynecology. There, patients were recovering from their surgeries and in some cases from the complications caused by, or that ensued after, those surgeries. Usually the medical and surgical specialties were kept apart, but administrators found that by merging them, they could amalgamate services and reduce duplication. However, that sometimes made for an uneasy juxtaposition of incompatible philosophies and personalities. The Medical approach involved subtleties such as the alchemy of cheicals and the passage of time. They discussed both the "big picture" and the minutiae of details and ideas and used delightful words and phrases, such as "angry rash," "integrity of the skin," "cardiac embarrassment," an injury to the heart muscle, or "defervescence," which referred to an overall deterioration in the patient's condition. The Medical docs were in it for the long haul, were satisfied with small gains and took the inevitable setbacks in stride. They knew they couldn't fix everything, but it was a darned interesting process to try a little of this and a little of that and see what happened.

On the other hand, surgeons were focused on the bottom line, in "cutting" to the chase, and in *outcomes*. They looked for opportunities to excise and resect (remove and chop) or suture and anastomize (sew and glue) and liked to fix the things they could and quickly became disinterested in the things they couldn't. Many had favourite nurses and flirted with them, whether they were attractive or not. There were always a few who lived up to their stereotype, like the surgeon who showed up one busy morning, needing help with a procedure he wanted to perform on my patient. "Hey, I'm putting a chest tube in Mr. Kanji," he said in an offhand manner. "He's got a pneumothorax and I may need a hand."

"And you would be . . . ?" I asked as I continued preparing my medications.

"Hi, I'm Vince, from Thoracic Surgery." He extended his hand.

"Hi, I'm Tilda, from Nursing," I said, mocking him ever so slightly. "I'll help you with that procedure as soon as I give the patient something for pain first."

"Oh, he won't be needing it. The way I work doesn't hurt a bit."

"But he's already in a lot of discomfort from his surgery."

"Don't worry, he'll be fine. I'm very fast."

I bet you are. "But, even so . . ." I recalled having read somewhere that "Pain is usually under-reported, under-ordered, under-administered, and thus under-treated." I couldn't bear to think of doing that procedure – which involved making a deep cut into the chest in between his ribs, inserting a large, thick plastic tube into his deflated lung, and applying strong suction pressure once it was in place – without local anaesthetic and a painkiller first.

"He won't need it," Vince said cheerfully, looking at his watch. "Can we get started?"

Oh, I get it. You don't want to wait while I get the keys and go to the narcotics cupboard for the drug. Then you'll have to wait a few minutes more for me to give it and for it to take effect.

"Don't worry," he cajoled. "I have superb technique." He patted me on the back. "None of my patients ever complain."

"That's because most of your patients are under general anaes-thetic."

"Aren't there any *nice* nurses around any more?" he teased, and I glared back at him.

Was it possible that he could really do such a smooth job that it wouldn't make a difference to the patient? Was I being over-conscientious? We stood on either side of the patient's bed and looked down at the man's emaciated and bony body. I decided not to be on my side or the doctor's, just the patient's. I tried to fly inside his mind, so I would know what to do.

"Hey, is this guy even conscious?" Vince asked.

The patient had grunted and moaned a few times while we stood there but didn't seem aware of us, of our conversation or its meaning. "Anyone can see he's in discomfort," I said, and it was true.

"Okay, go ahead, give him something if it'll make you feel better."

I ran out and came back quickly with the drug. "Until this takes effect, there's the sink," I teased him. He hadn't even washed his hands.

"You're a pretty tough cookie, aren't you?" he grinned, donning a sterile cap and gown.

I hung a small bag of saline with two milligrams of morphine injected into it, but he didn't like this slow method. "Push it in, fast," he ordered, but I told him no. "I have to give it this way."

"But it will take too long to take effect if you do it like that."

"Even so . . ." Every patient reacted differently to narcotics – to all painkillers, in fact. For some, a small dose was enough to treat severe pain. For others with milder pain, a larger dose had little effect. Soon, the morphine eased our patient and the procedure went smoothly, and just before Vince left he asked me out. But I turned him down because first of all, he was a jerk and second of all, it was around that time that I had reconnected with an old boyfriend I'd met in Israel. His name was Ivan Lewis and things were getting pretty serious between us.

UNFORTUNATELY, I DIDN'T ALWAYS speak up as assertively as I did that day. Once, after spending more than an hour on a complicated abdominal dressing that required rigorous sterile technique and deep internal packing, I had moved on to care for another patient when suddenly I heard an angry voice in the hall outside the previous patient's room.

"Where's a nurse? I need a nurse in here right away!"

I ran back to find one of the staff surgeons tearing away at the bandages I had just spent so much time putting in place. "I need to have a look at this incision," he barked, ripping away at the tape and gauze pads and leaving the wound exposed. "Who did this dressing?" he growled. I swore under my breath as I stood watching him make a mess of my work. The patient seemed a bit bewildered but pleased to have his doctor there. "Would someone bring me a fucking pair of scissors?" the doctor shouted, right in front of the patient, and then glared at me, clearly the someone he had in mind. I scurried off to hunt some down. It wasn't an easy thing to do as each hospital kept supplies in a different place and I was always going on a scavenger hunt.

"Grin and bear it." A nurse passing me in the hall saw I was upset. "We're nurses, aren't we?"

"Why do we have to take it?" I fumed.

"Don't let him get to you," she advised. "He makes everyone uptight, but he's a surgeon, you know. They get away with murder."

That remark made me giggle as I rushed back into the room, scissors in hand. But by then, the doctor was gone. He'd managed to remove the rest of the bandage by himself. The dirty gauze littered the bed and floor. The wound was left wide open. The patient's covers were thrown back and his gown was askew.

"How am I doing, nurse?" the patient looked up at me. "The doctor didn't mention."

"Your incision is healing nicely." I was steaming mad as I repacked the wound with sterile gauze and then cleaned up the mess. On the bedside table, beside the chart, I found a fancy pen the doctor had left behind. He'd used it to write in the chart. It had gold-coloured letters spelling out the name of a drug company. I did what anyone would do in that situation. I stole his pen.

THEN THERE CAME A NIGHT so crazy and chaotic, so stressful and upsetting, that by the end of that shift, I was ready to call it quits – being a nurse, I mean. I was sent to a medical surgical ward where I'd worked before, but this time, they put me in charge. In short order, I had to know everything about the medical condition of all of the thirty-two patients and be the one ultimately responsible for their nursing care. Luckily, Scott, the RPN, was on that night, and I knew from experience that I could count on him. However, Colleen, another RN, was also on and I knew from experience that I could not count on her. Skinny and low-energy and often in a bad mood, Colleen looked particularly disgruntled when she showed up late that night. She didn't greet me, but I caught up with her and re-introduced myself.

"Hi," I said with a fake smile. "I'm new," I added nervously.

"Hi, New. I noticed someone put you in charge."

"I mean, my name is Tilda. I'm from an agency, so it makes more sense for you to be in charge as you're staff here," I said. "You know the patients better than I do."

"Who said I wanted to be in charge? They obviously figure a university nurse is better for the job. Anyway, you're welcome to it. Enjoy!" She showed me a doctor's note. "Just to let you know. I hurt my back. I can't do any heavy lifting."

No lifting? Lifting was easy. The uplifting was the hard part.

Colleen went off to prepare medications for her patients and I sat down at the nurses' station beside Scott at a table covered with patient charts. "Colleen's got a chip on her shoulder," he explained, opening the box of doughnuts he'd brought in, "but she's a good nurse. Problem is, sometimes she's just not that into patient care."

What else is there, I wondered? "Mmm . . ." I murmured as if I understood.

"Colleen's the type that if she worked in a supermarket she'd prefer to handle the cash and bag groceries rather than deal with customers, you know what I mean? Anyway, relax, girlfriend, we'll manage." He passed me the box of doughnuts. "Here, have a 'tractor wheel.'" It was what he called the sugary, ridged crullers. "Or, a Boston Cream, if it doesn't make you think of draining an abscess."

I chose a plain glazed one. It was a wonder I ever even had an appetite at the hospital, but I usually did. Anyway, there was no more time to chat because I had just gotten word from the resident on call that we were receiving a new admission from the Emergency department. "Scott, you'd better get started with the vitals and the baths. After I finish transcribing the orders, I'll go around and do the IVs, dressing changes, the meds, and the peritoneal dialysis."

"Sounds like a plan. Don't worry, Tilda. There are only two patients who are PBS tonight and one guy coming in now who's HIBGIA." I waited for him to fill me in and he complied. "C'mon, girlfriend, get with the program. 'Pretty Bad Shape' and 'Had It Before, Got It Again.'"

"You'll have to keep a close eye on this new admission," the resident said, wheeling a stretcher into the ward. "He's a seventy-something homeless man with asthma and congestive heart failure."

Until I called Medical Records, I didn't even know his name was Mr. Fred Olsen. His chart was so heavy and in so many volumes that the porter brought it up from downstairs in a wheelchair. I went to see him and stood looking down at a poor, dirty person sprawled in the bed. His breathing was noisy and laboured and when I placed an oxygen saturation monitor on his finger to get a sense of his tissue perfusion, I got an abnormally low reading of 75 per cent, so I cranked up the oxygen concentration.

"If he deteriorates during the night," the resident said almost hopefully, "we'll be able to transfer him out to the ICU." The doctor's beeper rang and he had to run off, but I stayed behind with the patient. His oxygen mask hung loosely on his thin face and scraggly beard and I tightened it to fit better. I saw that he had soiled himself and so I went to get a basin of water, clean sheets, and a fresh gown. I got to work bathing him, all the while thinking about the multitude of equally pressing things that needed attending to. A man peeked into the room and asked to see the doctor. "He was just called away, but he'll be back in a few minutes. Is there a problem? Can I help you?" I came out into the hallway to talk to him.

"No offence, but you're just the . . ."

Yes, what am I? I dare you to say it. He changed his tack.

"How is my mother doing?" he asked politely. "She seems confused."

Which one was she? I ran through my notes to refresh my memory. Luckily, I had read her chart. "Confusion is common after a stroke. It may improve with time. It's still too early to say."

"What? Mother had a stroke? Why didn't anyone tell us?"

The man followed after me as I went to the nurses' station and reviewed her chart, but there was nothing much to tell him about his mother as the doctor hadn't yet examined her. The CT scan done in the Emergency department showed she had suffered a stroke and that lots of blood work had been drawn and other tests performed, but the results were still pending. Since I had nothing more to tell him and about twenty other places I had to be at that moment, I turned away from his anxious face and whizzed past him. I couldn't spare a moment even to help him prop his mother up in bed so that she could sip a cup of tea. Colleen was nowhere to be found and Scott needed help with a patient, a forty-year-old man who that afternoon had swallowed paint thinner in a suicide attempt and was now vomiting blood. I showed Scott how to irrigate the patient's naso-gastric tube with saline and left him with that and went out to the large group of family members waiting outside the door. "How was Salim before this happened?" I asked them. There was so little information in the chart and a considerable language barrier between us.

"He was good, very good, thank you, miss." They bowed slightly, grateful for my concern.

"Was he unhappy about something?"

"Oh, no, nurse, he wasn't unhappy. Salim is such a very happy person."

"What led him to do such a thing?"

"Well, he lost his job at the paint factory and his wife left him and took the kids back to India."

"Oh, I see." Now I had too much information. I smiled at their old granny who was blowing kisses to me. She was hobbling around with a cane and looked like she'd just flown in from the streets of Calcutta with her black teeth, dusty feet in sandals, wearing a flowing brown sari with a veil that trailed down her back and nose ring in the shape of a daisy. She smiled at me, put her palms together, and bowed. I bowed to her in return and then went to find her a wheelchair. Since I couldn't find one, I put her on a swivel chair from the nurses' station and she blew more kisses at me as her grandchildren gave her rides, wheeling her up and down the halls. Just then I heard Colleen call out, "Come quick!" and I rushed into the room and saw a mini-geyser of blood spurting out of her patient's groin. He had undergone an angiogram that day and the site where a huge needle had been placed was gushing. I grabbed a pile of sterile gauze, reached down into the folds of his belly and slapped it on the spot. I pressed my full weight upon it to staunch the blood. I put Colleen in place to keep pressure on the spot until the bleeding stopped and I went off to page the surgeon.

I spent the entire night running from crisis to crisis. In between, I was answering the telephone, speaking with families, ordering drugs from the pharmacy, filling out forms, paging doctors, ordering trays from the kitchen, restocking cupboards, cleaning rooms. It was well after four o'clock in the morning and I had yet to begin to make a dent in my charting, but I decided to check on the homeless man one more time. I turned the light away so as not to wake the other patient in the room who was snoring lightly. At first I thought Mr. Olsen was asleep, too, but upon closer examination, I saw that he was dead. Now, there would be a slew of paperwork, a call to the morgue, and, once his bed was vacated, the possibility to get a new admission in his place. "Well, at least it's one less to worry about," the resident said, coming up to stand beside me at the patient's bedside, and I hate to admit it but I had just had the exact same thought.

It's almost over, I told myself as the day shift began to arrive. *This is my last shift, my last night as a nurse.* I was throwing in the towel. (I would have thrown in my cap, too, if I wore one in the first place.) I sat down to collect my scattered thoughts as I prepared to hand over to the oncoming charge nurse. I went through them one by one. "Mr. X . . . wound still inflamed, spiked a temp last night . . . Mrs. Y, slept well, good pain control . . . Mr. Z . . . less nausea but urine output still low." Then I came to a report about a patient I couldn't recall. "Mr. Henderson," I said, reading the note slowly. "Low blood pressure. Cerebral hemorrhage, unconscious, neck fracture . . ." Who was this? How could I not know about a patient, especially one this sick? I saw Colleen snickering and whispering to her day shift friends, who looked over at me and laughed. She had set me up! Some jokes are meant to provoke laughter and others to provoke embarrassment and this was of the latter type. But hadn't I been warned? *Nurses eat their* *young.* Unfortunately, I had never learned how you avoided becoming someone's live bait.[*]

Just as I was leaving, the nurse manager came over to ask me to stay for a few hours of overtime. "We're dangerously short-staffed. How 'bout it, Tilda?"

"Sorry. No can do," I told her curtly without even offering a reason. *Let me outta here. Let me put an end to this nightmare.* But still, it was not to be. As I tried to leave again, a nurse shouted from the medication room. "Call the Mounties! The narcotics count is off." She'd said it like a joke, but it was a serious situation and no one could leave until we reconciled the count. The morphine tallied, as did the Codeine and the Dilaudid, but two vials of Demerol were missing. As the nurse in charge, I was held responsible and had to fill out an incident report. Unaccounted-for narcotics was never taken lightly and I knew this report would become a permanent part of my record. Again, I saw Colleen smirking as she left. I didn't know if she had had anything to do with it – whether she was a possible user or simply a troublemaker – and I didn't even care at that point.

"Rough night?" said the nurse manager, coming back over to me.

I shot her a murderous glance but my rudeness didn't dissuade her from reaching out to me.

"Come to my office. Let's have a chat."

I shook my head because I knew if I spoke, I would cry, and if I cried, I would lose it altogether. "I'll come," I told her, "but I have nothing to say." Yet the moment she sat down opposite me and gave me her undivided attention, I spilled my guts and told her everything. Not just about that horrific night and the homeless man who had died alone and the bleeding groin and Colleen, but about Buddy, too, and about the suppurating wound, and the patient who called me Maggie and about how impossible, frustrating, and

---

[*] However, it did make me recall my father's old joke about the cannibal who was eating a clown and stopped to complain that something, "tasted funny."

soul-destroying it was to be a nurse. She listened to me, nodding
her head from time to time. I expected her to tell me to toughen up
and get better at my skills and at organizing myself, but she said
none of that. What she did say surprised me. "You have to learn
how to get in and how to get out." You have to care, she explained,
but not too much, or it will interfere with your ability to be effective. "Fix what you can and leave the rest. Some things you can't
make better." I must have looked dubious. "I know it sounds
harsh," she said, "but it's the kindest thing. The most helpful."

"I may be having a nervous breakdown," I warned her, holding
my head in my hands.

"You're exhausted," she said kindly.

Yes, there are times when sleep is the only solution.

6

THINKING LIKE A NURSE

The "All-Day-Breakfast" must have been invented for people who work at night because nothing tastes better than poached eggs, buttered toast, and hot coffee in a greasy spoon diner, in the late afternoon after an entire day lost to sleep. That horrible night shift, I had intended to call it quits, but with sleep and food so fine, my outlook improved. I decided to stay, after all. Besides, I needed nursing more than nursing needed me. Fortunately, around that time – it was 1988 – there was a sea change in the job market and hospital officials decided that instead of layoffs, more nurses were, in fact, needed. Headhunters went scouting, offering incentives of sign-on bonuses and education subsidies. Opportunities abounded. "Recruitment and retention" suddenly became the new buzzwords, making it sound like a military operation.

But before I had a chance to apply for any of those jobs, my mother's condition worsened and I was faced with a difficult decision. Her doctor in the hospital called me to come in. We walked together down the corridor. "Your mother has pneumonia," he said gently. "Her condition has been severely debilitated for some time. Did she ever discuss her wishes with you?"

My mother had told me exactly what she wanted, but I never really believed I would be in a position to have to carry it out. "I don't know," I lied.

"The burden of treatment must be weighed against possible benefits so as to avoid unnecessary suffering," he said in a kind but formal way.

"What are the choices?"

"To withhold further treatments, discontinue feeding, and wait and see. Or . . ." He paused before option number two. "To transfer her to the ICU, institute life support measures, and then wait and see."

I told him I would think it over. I hung up the phone and went into the cafeteria. Even though I wasn't the least bit hungry, I bought a butterscotch sundae in a small plastic cup that had a tiny wooden paddle for a spoon. I thought about using that little oar to push off from shore and row out into the high seas in order to get as far away from all of this as I could. I understood the choices before me, and I wondered how I would feel after each fateful one. *Do me in, she'd told me. Find a way.* From the age of six, I knew my mother's wishes, but now would I have the courage to carry them out?

I went back up to her room. She had a fever and I sat beside her and placed a cool cloth on her forehead. A medical student came in to take blood. He poked at her arms that were covered in bruises from previous needle attempts, but soon gave up and left. My mother was in her fifties, but she looked eighty. She no longer responded to the music on the radio I played for her and now, barely spoke.

A nurse came in and took her vital signs but there was nothing vital about my mother's grey pallor or her raspy breathing. When the nurse left, I leaned down close to my mother to hear if there was any last message, but her breath had an unpleasant, medicinal smell that made me pull away. She looked at me but I don't think she saw me.

"You have a difficult decision to make," the doctor said when he came back into the room. "Your mother is critically ill. Again, the choices are to transfer her to the ICU and put her on life support or keep her here and focus on her comfort. Did she ever discuss the matter with you?"

"Yes, she did," I told him. "She told me many years ago, and again on many occasions." I said I knew she wouldn't want to go to the ICU because whatever they might be able to offer her there, she would never again be able to sing and that was all she really wanted. The doctor agreed that a palliative approach was wise, but we decided to continue with antibiotics and feeding. I guess I wasn't entirely ready to let go yet.

The nurses kept her clean and comfortable. They talked to her and caressed her and stayed even closer by her side, offering her the loving kindness that I hadn't been able to for years. I couldn't bear to visit her. A few days later, a nurse called to tell me the news. "Your mother has improved. Her fever is down." The doctor was also impressed. "Given her premorbid condition, I didn't expect a recovery, but her superb pulmonary function pulled her through. She's got the respiratory reserve of an athlete with huge tidal volumes. It is extraordinary how she sings little tunes for the nurses at a moderate volume but her speech remains barely audible."

"She always said breathing was the most important thing."

"Now that your mother has recovered," the doctor said, "we will have to fill out the papers for her to be placed in a chronic care facility."

But her recovery was shortlived. Within a few weeks, the pneumonia returned and this time ravaged her even more. One afternoon Pearl met me at the nurses' station, her face glistening with tears. "She's gone." She wiped her eyes with her fingers and hugged me. "And I say, good for her! Praise the Lord!"

I could hardly believe it had finally happened. She had been dying for years but this time it was for real. "Why do you say that, Pearl?"

"She's in the arms of the Lord. Her suffering is over."

"Her life was sad," I lamented.

"Yes, but she was saved," Pearl exclaimed. "She took the Lord Jesus into her heart just in time, before she died. Read Psalms: 'Alas for those who cannot sing, but die with all their music in them.'"

"Who was she, Pearl? Did you ever get to know her?"

"I did! I loved that woman. I do! I loved her like my chile."

I loved her that way, too, even when I was a child myself. She was my first patient and a gentle soul who adored beautiful music but cried when she heard it. She adored elegant clothes, but rarely wore them. She admired great books, but never read them. I had missed her all my life and now that she was dead, suddenly, I no longer missed her.

My three brothers were at the funeral, but we didn't speak much. I could see that Robbie was mentally not well. "I made you take care of me," he said. "I was very disturbed. Do not underestimate the very-ness of that disturbed." I tried to put my arm around him, but he pulled away. My other two brothers seemed happy. They would be okay.

"I'm sorry for your loss," the Rabbi said to us. "We can only hope she's in a better place now."

"It couldn't be much worse," said Stephen under his breath.

The Rabbi spoke of her magnificent voice and her thwarted career as an opera singer. He told of her dignity and the courage with which she met her challenges. I sat there, squelching my memories of all the harsh things I'd said, the rough way I'd handled her at times, and the promises I'd broken. I thought of the tender nursing care I'd given to other people, yet the only patient for whom I couldn't muster sufficient compassion was my mother. I sat there and tried hard not to think about the one long black velvet glove with pearl buttons that she wore when she sang. I had found it among her belongings and had searched all night for the mate.

I was in my late twenties and grief seemed familiar to me now, this second time around, mourning my other parent's death. I knew that the sharp pain would eventually subside, that it would always be lodged inside me, more bearable with time. For a few days I was tempted to follow my old escape route, underground into the subway, but a newer, stronger core within me was developing and I made the decision to go forward with my life. I decided to accept a position at Toronto General Hospital in the Intensive Care Unit. It was the same hospital where I had gone with my mother to her appointments with the neurologist Dr. DeGroot, and to my father's various doctors. It was the hospital where I had first worked as a candystriper and then in the patients' lending library, distributing novels and magazines. Now, its Department of Nursing was offering a critical care course and upon its successful completion, a staff position in the ICU. It had only ten beds at that time but there were plans to expand.

The ICU was dark and cramped with two patients in each room. In fact, one room was located so far from the nurses' station and was so poorly lit that it was called the Cave. Needless to say, no one wanted to work there. There was a hushed, tense atmosphere in the ICU, punctuated by the frequent beeping, buzzing, and ringing of machines in each room. Attached to the equipment, the patients were unconscious, lying stretched out on huge beds. The nurses all wore green scrubs, the walls and countertops were pale green, and in my imagination, there was a ghoulish green hue on some of the patients' faces. The place made me queasy. I jumped up a few times during the nights before work, always afraid I would sleep in. The ICU environment scared me, and the prospect of taking care of critically ill patients terrified me, yet I think that's why I chose it. I wanted to face what I was most afraid of and master it. I'll never forget my first day and how Laura, the charge nurse, greeted me. "Welcome to the House of Horrors," she said with a grim laugh. She was pretty, but I could tell that her good looks didn't matter to her. In spite of my fear, I couldn't help but feel thrilled to be part of the ICU team, facing the incredible challenges of bringing people who were on the brink of death, back to life.

I immersed myself into my work – caring for patients with the most catastrophic, life-threatening illnesses imaginable. There were people recovering from massive surgery to their chest or abdomen and the doctors there were even starting to perform liver and lung transplants. There were cases of cardiogenic shock, septic shock, and multi-system failure, where more than one of the major organs was malfunctioning or had shut down altogether. Doctors were on-call at all times, but each nurse was assigned one or two patients at most and assumed complete responsibility for all of the nursing care that patient needed. Doctors came and went, but the nurses always stayed close to the patients and their families.

There was so much to learn, so many numbers and formulas to memorize and complex concepts to grasp, that for the first few weeks, I operated on a strictly need-to-know basis. I couldn't absorb anything extra. Everything seemed urgent and top priority and I wasn't always efficient enough to get technical jobs done fast enough. For example, I often spent an inordinate amount of time sorting out the tubes, wires, and lines that always bunched up around the patient. The nurses called it "spaghetti" and invariably one of them would sense my frustration and arrive on the scene to help me out. (It was a task akin to disentangling necklaces that become inexplicably and impossibly intertwined from merely lying in a jewellery box.) Those experienced nurses knew lots of tricks with their hands, like how to use gravity or negative pressure to get fluids to flow in or out of the body and how to apply traction or leverage to position patients more comfortably in bed. They often jerry-rigged various pieces of equipment to get them to work the way they liked and some even kept a screwdriver and a surgical clamp (which they used as a wrench when needed) in their pockets.

Within the larger team of nurses, there were six of us whom I ended up working with closely for many years. We were dubbed "Laura's Line," but if we had been the "Spice Girls," Laura would have been pungent Garlic; Frances, heart-warming Cinnamon; Tracy, elemental, essential Salt; Justine, spicy Cayenne Pepper; Nicky, sweet Maple Sugar; and I, Coriander, an acquired taste that grows on you over time, or so I've been told.

Even back then, Laura was a paradox. Brusque and sarcastic toward doctors, demanding and critical of other nurses, irreverent and dismissive toward administrators and politicians, Laura was at all times exquisitely kind and exceedingly gentle with her patients. She was intelligent and very well read, yet she had little respect for formal education. Patients loved her, but Laura prided herself on never getting too attached to them.

"One thing, I can tell you," Laura said to me early on. We were sitting in the staff lounge during a coffee break, and she stretched out on the couch, her arms behind her head. "The personal stuff is highly overrated. I never get emotionally involved with my patients."

"How can you care for people and not have a relationship with them?" I asked in dismay.

"I've taken care of a lot of patients over the years and never felt I had to get to *know* them," she shot back. "Give me a break, Tilda! There are too many of them and they're too sick and there isn't enough time or enough of us."

"Haven't you noticed how it means so much to patients when nurses get emotionally involved with them?"

"Patients also tend to favour nurses who give them the right medications on time, too!"

Laura showed little deference to doctors. She addressed them all by their first names and when a weekend was coming up, she not-too subtly suggested that they treat the team to bagels and cream cheese or pastries. And if a resident wanted to perform a procedure on her patient and asked her to bring him sterile drapes, an angiocath, a scalpel, and a pair of forceps, Laura didn't miss a beat. "Do you want fries with that?" she'd ask. When the doctor finished the procedure and if he should turn to walk out of the room, she would call him right back to clean up the mess of bloody towels, used swabs, and especially "sharps" – the needles, wires, and blades – he'd left behind. "Why should she clean up his mess or risk her safety handling things he had used?" she'd ask him. And just before she released him, if he had written a slew of orders in the chart, she stopped him. "Whoa, there. You can't split without discussing those with me. I'm in charge of this patient's care." Eventually, she set him free and he would scurry off.

She spoke in the same way to senior staff doctors. If one of the specialists asked Laura about her patient, she might say, "That depends," not looking up from whatever she was doing. "Tell me who you are first. If you're from Neurology, then he's improving. If you're from Cardiology, he's stable, but if you're from the liver team, he's in a bad way."

Once I asked Laura about my patient's Central Venous Pressure. "Where do the doctors want the CVP to be?" I asked her. By then I understood the various manipulations that we could make with fluids and medications to affect the heart's functioning. "Where do *they* want it?" she shot back. "Where do *you* think it should be? Don't just follow orders. Think it through yourself."

Frances was the softie in our group, and I don't know how I would have survived those first few scary weeks in the ICU if she hadn't been there. She always made herself available to me and was at my side the first time I had to suction a patient, something we had to do to remove secretions from the lungs. He was on a ventilator and had a breathing tube. "This will make you cough," I told him timidly, and he nodded his assent for me to proceed. "I know it's uncomfortable, but afterwards you'll feel better," I explained unconvincingly. I hesitated and tried to steel myself to perform this procedure that I knew would be unpleasant for him. "Here," said Frances, "let me show you." She did it smoothly and the patient nodded his appreciation of her more confident style.

"Smile," Frances said to me afterwards, and I did, broadly, falsely. "That's better. At least try to look like you're having fun, then maybe you will."

I don't know exactly how she did it, but Frances made patients feel she was doing things *for* them and *with* them, not *to* them. She saw the patients' room as their personal space that she entered with their permission. And although Frances could perform advanced and high-tech skills as well as anyone, it was providing care and comfort measures that she most prided herself on. "Never neglect the *basics*," she explained to me on many occasions. "You have to keep the mouth clean and the skin moisturized." She also meant the turning and the lifting, the rubbing and the massaging, keeping patients' hair washed and tidy, trimming beards, cutting toenails, removing wax from ears, rubbing mineral oil onto the soles of scaly feet, and at all times, keeping patients clean and comfortable on smooth, fresh sheets. These were the dreary, menial jobs, the "custodial care" that many university-educated nurses assumed a degree would exempt them from. Yet, Frances performed them like they were almost sacred tasks and regarded them at times as having even greater importance than sophisticated procedures. "It's when you are doing these things that you can assess the condition of your patient's skin, their oxygenation, and pain and so on. Some nurses think doing these things is beneath them, but I don't and never will," she said.

One day, to my surprise, Frances called upon me to help her. She was caring for an elderly Chinese man who was dying. With the family's consent, I joined the intimate circle around his bed. Frances instructed me to place warm towels all over the patient, with a few extra around his neck, as this was part of the Chinese custom of keeping the body warm. And when she noticed that the family was ill at ease and unsure of what to say or do, she guided them. "Tell him you are here," Frances said, motioning them to move in closer around the bed. "Say the names of each person here today with him. Let him hear the sounds of your voices."

"Can he hear us?" they asked.

Frances nodded. "You may not get a response, but talk to him anyway."

"We don't want to disturb him." They were afraid and drew back.

"This is hard for you, but he is peaceful. He's comfortable." Frances let down the side rails so they could be even closer if they wanted. "It's okay. Hold his hand. That will make him feel loved and secure." She gave them a cloth to wipe his brow, a moist swab for his mouth, and I could see their fear lessen as they did these small actions. When he began to take his last breaths, Frances put her arms across their backs. She stayed with them until the last heartbeat, the last breath.

For me, it was fascinating to watch how a person died, organ by organ. The technology of the ICU exposed everything. All the body's secrets were revealed. I watched the kidneys shut down, the blood pressure diminish, the heart slow down to a wavy, then horizontal green line, the irregular breathing pattern of the lungs mapped out on the ventilator screen, the incremental diminishment of oxygen to the tissues, and all the while, the gradual loss of consciousness. I watched death happen and saw how it could be measured, charted, documented – even *manipulated*. It was no wonder, in fact, that when Frances shut off the cardiac monitor, the family took that flip of a switch to be the moment of death.

"Is he gone?" they asked and her "yes" was as gentle as possible. They asked her to please open the windows so that their father's spirit could escape into the afterworld, but Frances explained that that was not possible because the hospital windows could not be opened. That distressed them, but there was nothing that could be done. Then the family left and I helped Frances wash the body and remove all the tubes, lines, and machines. All the while that we worked, she kept a quiet, almost reverential silence. Then she brought the family back in so that they could spend time with the body, pay their last respects, and chant prayers.

"Salt-of-the-earth" Tracy was tall, skinny, utterly unflappable, and at times, inscrutable. She had an uncanny – almost spooky – way of appearing just when you needed her the most, without your even asking. And she had a respectful way of helping, so that you felt she was assisting you, not coming to your rescue because you were freaking out and not coping with the crisis yourself. Tracy said little and in fact was so quiet and serious that occasionally when she cracked a joke, it snuck up on me. I was sitting with her in the staff lounge one day and she was telling me about a patient of hers who had lung cancer. "I was giving her a bath," Tracy said. "She seemed fine, but all of a sudden, out of the blue, she burst into tears."

"What happened?" I gasped.

"She told me she was afraid the surgeons didn't get it all and that she might die."

"What did you say?" I asked, wondering what I would have said.

"I said, 'C'mon, knock it off, don't be such a crybaby. Put on a happy face.'"

"You said that to her?!"

"No, you doofus. There was nothing to say. I just sat with her and held her hand while she cried."

She said it as if it were nothing, but it seemed to me something fairly important.

In contrast to Tracy and her subtle manner, Justine was known to be a spicy chili pepper and not just because of her flaming red hair. She had a fiery tongue and could be brutally honest, but most people took it from her – even patients' families – without ques-tion, because she was totally fair-minded and completely without malice. She enjoyed working in the ICU but saw its limitations. She believed we often went too far with some patients and decried the fact that we didn't know most of our patients' wishes. She was con-vinced that if they could speak for themselves, many would refuse the extreme measures we were offering them. Even though these were delicate situations, Justine's humour could be outrageous. Once, I went over to chat with her and she casually mentioned with a wicked grin that her patient was about to be transferred out. I looked at the number of pumps and machines in the room and the ominous numbers and abnormal waveforms on the monitor screens. "Transferred out? You mean he's going home? How?"

"Yeah, he's going home all right – in a jar. He'll be transferred out to the Eternal Care Centre. You know, the Celestial Discharge Unit."

It was a horrible joke, but what a relief it was to laugh. Justine provided that opportunity for all of us on many occasions and sometimes for patients as well. "You're a Scorpio?" she said to one young man she was caring for, noting the date of birth on his chart. "Hey, me too! Scorpios rock!" As anxious and worried about their loved one as a family might be, Justine always managed to get a laugh out of them. Walking past her patient's room one day, I was shocked to hear her say to a family who was barraging her with questions and demands, "Stop it, you guys! You're driving me crazy!" Rather than being affronted by her, I saw how she put them at ease. After all, they must have figured, how bad could it be if the nurse was joking around?

As for Nicky (pure maple sugar), it was probably not a good idea for us to work together because we chatted far too much. We gossiped about boyfriends, travel plans, and forbidden liaisons and rendezvous between certain doctors and nurses that only we knew about. We talked as we bathed our patients. Nicky would wash one leg, and I, the other. She soaped up one armpit while I rinsed off the other. She took temperatures and I recorded the blood pressures. One patient moved his head from side to side watching our routine and as ill as he was, couldn't help but laugh at our antics.

As for me, I thought of myself as coriander, a herb my father used liberally in his cooking. It has a flavour that most either love or decidedly, not. My father claimed it was a delicate yet hardy plant with both a sweet and bitter flavour, and in the proper growing conditions, it would flourish. Coriander, he explained, had special properties because it was neither exclusively wild nor domestic; it was a "cultivated weed." I was coriander in those days in the ICU where I felt I was finally flourishing in the proper environment. It was a place where I also had the opportunity to explore many different ways of being a nurse.

I studied all of the nurses I worked with, adopting the traits I liked. I was in awe of Laura, who engendered such affection and confidence in her patients. There were others like her who were no less caring even as they kept their emotions intact. I admired Frances and Nicky and other nurses like them who *did* connect personally with patients, yet I often saw, in private moments, how it took its toll on them. I longed to be as calm and focused as Tracy. As for Justine – what a pistol! I hoped one day to have the courage she had to stand up for what she believed was right – whether it was advocating for patients or for nurses – and to find a way, as she did, to use humour to make people feel better.

I wonder if any of the nurses suspected that I was "spying" on them, listening in to their conversations with patients and watching how they handled difficult situations. I admired how some always managed to find something hopeful or positive to say, even when the patient was getting worse or dying. Some nurses took such care with seemingly small things, for example, ensuring to cover up parts of the body they weren't washing to keep the person warm and unexposed or warming up a metal bedpan before putting it in place underneath the patient – and how others didn't take or make the time to do these things. Some noticed even minute things, such as the discomfort caused by a bit of plastic jutting out from the IV tubing. They would fold up a pillowcase and place that softness between the plastic and the patient's skin. They would ensure the urinary catheter was anchored so that it wouldn't pull and they would gently ask a family's permission to remove jewellery, especially a wedding ring, with soap or Vaseline, knowing very well that soon the fingers would swell, making it impossible to remove without cutting it off. I watched nurses who accompanied families into the ICU for their first visit and how they caught them when they drew away, fell back, or even fainted, shocked at the sight of their loved one's condition. Some nurses knew how to actually help the family *befriend* those scary machines. This is what we do in the ICU, they explained to them. It's what's normal here. Once those machines have served their purpose, they will be removed, but for now, they are needed.

They could make the most extreme situations seem ordinary in a way that calmed the patient. "There's blood pouring out of your rectum," I heard a nurse say to his patient as if that was an everyday occurrence. Later he told him, "Your heart is going in and out of a wacky rhythm, but I'm giving you a medication in your IV and we'll get it settled down." I went over afterward to tell him that I liked the way he'd handled the crisis, but he brushed the compliment aside and waved me away.

And I don't think any nurse ever forgets the first time they participated in a "code," a cardiac or respiratory arrest. That's when you truly feel you are an essential member of the team. Finally, in the ICU, I wasn't just standing by while the rest of the team sprang into action, everyone knowing what to do. I became one of the ones who ran in to help. Undeniably, we were having an adrenalin rush as we came together, our hands swarming over the patient, doing chest compressions, giving electric shocks, drawing blood, and pushing medications. Often we didn't even know if we were keeping someone alive or staving off death, but in those moments it didn't matter. (Perhaps it amounted to the same thing, but it implied a different mindset.) We were united in our efforts and if there were times that we were even grooving on that high and feeling so heroic and powerful, who of us would admit it?

Soon, I, too, could read the subtle clues and speak the insider language. If I started a shift and saw the crash cart wasn't in its storage corner, I searched for the room where there was a "busy" or "sick" patient, a patient in trouble who was "crashing." Coming into a patient's room and seeing ECG strips spewed out of the monitor, trailing all over the floor, curling up like party streamers, meant the patient had likely been having irregular heartbeats, called "arrhythmias." If the patient was on "bug drugs," I knew that antibiotics had been instituted and likely "tropes," too, which were inotropes, drugs, like Dopamine or Levophed, used to raise the blood pressure when it had dropped dangerously low. "Going travelling" meant transporting your patient to a test in another part of the hospital – no simple matter, considering how unstable they were and all the equipment they were attached to, including the portable "zapper," which was the defibrillator and all the "Christmas trees," the ringing, dinging, flashing IV pumps on either side of a patient.

But there were moments, after I got over my awe at it all, that I wondered, was I nursing the patient or the machines? Was I caring for the body in the bed or an electrophysiological representation of bodily functions on a monitor screen? There were many hours when my attention was entirely given over to the gadgets and gizmos of chrome, metal, glass, and plastic, as much as, if not more than, to the patient. I couldn't always bring the two together. It was Laura who got me thinking about these things. She fixed her level gaze on the patient first and the machines second. "That's where the truth is," she told me, nodding at a patient in the bed. "Don't believe everything you see up there," she waved at the cardiac monitor. "Hey, Tilda, watch this." She jumped up and down beside the monitor to create "artifact," making the screen imitate ventricular fibrillation, a lethal heart rhythm. We'd all seen her occasionally give a little kick or punch to a malfunctioning IV pump and get it started up again, buzzing happily back at work. "Oh, I believe in the sanctity of life, all right," Laura said one day after morning rounds, "but I don't worship technology. Take temperatures, for example. We measure them by mouth, under the arm, in the tympanic membrane of the ear, or in the rectum. We use mercury, water pressure, electronic pulsation, or a thermo-dilution catheter in a patient's pulmonary artery. But most nurses can feel their patient's forehead and tell if there's a fever."

Frances agreed. "It's true. Sometimes I touch the patient, take a guess at his temperature, and then measure it. I'm always accurate within a few tenths of a degree." Nicky and I looked over at Tracy, who didn't say anything. We had both seen Tracy predict a fever before the temperature even began to rise. She had a preternatural ability to know exactly what was going on with her patients long before the machines proved her right.

They were incredible nurses and the ICU provided perfect conditions in which to do our work.

"If only the nurses on the floor were as good as you ICU nurses," a doctor said to me one day with a huge sigh of exasperation. It was late afternoon and we were sitting at the nurses' station catching up on our charting. He was a third-year resident who was enjoying his ICU rotation. "The nurses on the floor don't know as much as you ICU nurses."

"It's not fair to compare them to us in our ideal conditions," I explained. "There aren't enough nurses on the floor and their workloads are impossible."

"But they don't even look at lab results. They don't know what's going on with their patients."

"They have no time, they're just trying to keep up." It hadn't been that long ago that I had worked on the floor myself and I well remembered how many times I'd left at the end of a shift feeling frustrated and discouraged. My work had fallen so short of my ideals that my ideals began to seem impossible. I had felt at the mercy of others, at everyone's beck and call, and powerless against whatever might be thrown at me. Nurses were often pitted against each other, even sabotaged one another, and were stressed and unhappy. But here in the ICU, nurses had a feeling of empowerment and a sense of their capacity to take action. We expressed our opinions vocally, sometimes even vociferously. None of us hesitated to do whatever was required to make things better. All nurses had a right to work like this and every patient had a right to receive care in a respectful, healthy environment, didn't they? Yet, that wasn't always the case. It was only when I got to the ICU that I finally experienced the possibility of mastery. Mastery was within my grasp.

COFFEE BREAKS WERE a respected and inviolable tradition in the
ICU. The nurses all took turns covering for each other so that we
could get away for even a few minutes. At first, I refused to leave,
saying I needed to stay behind to catch up. "No matter how busy
it is, you have to take a break," said Justine, that first day, herding
me out the door. "The work here is never done," said Frances
pulling me along by my arm. "You have to pace yourself." By then,
Laura had already left for her break, taking a longer, circuitous
route down the back stairs so she could avoid walking past the
room where the worried families waited.

In the cafeteria, we sat and watched Justine over at the menu
board, removing the decimal places so that the price of the lunch
special shot up from $5.95 to $595. We could hear her griping to
the head cook: "Does the World Health Organization know what
prices you're charging for this slop?" He pointed to a posted notice
that the cafeteria would soon be closed to make way for the more
profitable Subway, Burger King, and Pizza Hut chains. "The forces
of globalization strike again," Justine said, shaking her head.
"Retrenchment is in the works, too, I bet. What's your union say
about all this?"

"The hospital management promised us jobs," the cook said,
stirring a huge vat of soup.

"Ahh, I get it." She came back to explain to us. "They'll get the
pastry chefs to bathe patients so they can get rid of us 'expensive'
nurses. You'll see. That's the plan in the works."

Her worry was not unfounded. We knew from experience that
the hospital management didn't always value the work of skilled,
educated nurses, but at least we had Justine on our side, fighting
for our rights – and our jobs – if they became threatened once again.

EVERY MORNING THE ENTIRE TEAM – the staff doctor, the residents,
the nurse manager, the charge nurse, the patient's nurse, and a whole
range of other professionals, including the dietician and pharmacist,
the physiotherapist, and respiratory therapist – gathered outside
each patient's room to discuss the plan of treatment. The resident
presented a summary of the patient's medical history and current

condition and then the nurse highlighted particular problems identified in his or her morning assessment. Then the interesting part ensued – the debates. We looked at X-rays together and discussed the patient's fluid balance and whether or not the patient was in overload or in fact needed extra fluid. We might review the reasons for performing a lumbar puncture, weigh the risks and benefits of transporting an unstable patient for a CT scan, or consider the merits of various antibiotics. And always, there were complex dilemmas that we faced, such as whether to perform resuscitations on patients with multiple organ dysfunction even with the documented low success rate. Is this a futile practice? someone might ask, and we would all get an opportunity to express and explore our views. Morning rounds were like the Town Hall gatherings of philosophers in Ancient Greece. Questions were posed and discussions raged about great mysteries of the universe. Everyone had a say and all voices were heard and valued.

At the end of each twelve-hour shift, it was time to hand over our patients, and all the information we knew about them, to the oncoming nurse. Handover was a form of storytelling and some nurses were known for their engaging, even entertaining delivery, all the while still giving a comprehensive and organized report.[*] One nurse even had the hockey game on the radio and stopped to cheer when her team scored. I learned to give a decent, organized report and luxuriated afterward in the feeling of release of a weight of tension so palpable I was certain I had to be a few pounds lighter. When I got home, I was exhausted but elated, too, from a day intense with thinking, doing, feeling, and seeing so much.

ONE MORNING after I'd been working in the ICU for almost a year, the nurse in charge came over to tell me she'd assigned me the sickest patient. He had been admitted the night before into the room we

---

[*] I'll never forget the nurse who had a most disconcerting habit of repeatedly gesturing or pointing to the parts on my body that she was referring to on the patient's body such as the internal jugular IV site on my neck or the bowel obstruction on my abdomen. I didn't like it one bit.

called the Cave. She was paying me two compliments: I was being entrusted with the most unstable patient, and therefore the most challenging one, and I was expected to work independently. The rest of the team would not be as readily available, but of course would come running in an emergency. I went in and got to work. My patient was a sixty-five-year-old man, two days post abdominal surgery, who had developed subsequent complications of bleeding and infections. He had so many tubes, drains, ivs, and incisions that one nurse had drawn a map and labelled everything to help others navigate around the patient's body. Another nurse had thought to demarcate the area of bleeding around his incision with a permanent marker so that we could all keep an eye on its possible spread. I started off by searching for a flicker of the person, beginning with the neurological part of my head-to-toe nursing assessment. He was unconscious, but I spoke to him anyway. I listened to his heart and lungs and suctioned him efficiently. Justine came by to see how I was doing. She handed me a blood culture result on my patient and updated me on the latest tiff she'd had with the laboratory technicians. It seems she had told them her name was "Chi Chi" so they wouldn't be able to find her, *that nurse with the attitude*, and when they asked for her first name, she said, of course, "It's Chi." I saw that I could take care of everything for my patient and also laugh at her silly joke, too. Justine suddenly recalled the reason she'd come down to visit me in the Cave. "Oh, by the way, your patient is growing *filamentos fungus* in his blood," she chuckled. "I think I ordered that once in a Mexican restaurant." On the basis of that report, I spoke with the doctor and we changed the antibiotic to one that was sensitive to the particular organism growing in the blood culture.

"Your family is here," I told my patient as I beckoned them to come in. His wife and two grown-up children were shocked at the sight of their father, intubated, unresponsive, his face swollen, his entire body bloated. They couldn't bear to look at him and instead stared up at the monitor. I had the feeling the children almost envied me that I could do things for their father that they wished they knew how to do. I knew things about their father that they did not, such as his lab values and what they meant, how much urine he was producing and if he had called out for them during a moment of need. When he suddenly started coughing and his oxygen saturation plummeted from 99 per cent to 70 per cent, they jumped up and looked to me to fix the problem. I acted quickly and smoothly to extract a tenacious mucous plug lodged deep in his bronchus, all the while reassuring them and the patient, too.

"Good work, Tilda," one of the ICU doctors said as he passed by the room, and the family looked pleased I was their father's nurse.

"I'll take good care of him and you can call anytime," I re-assured them as they were leaving.

By the end of the day his blood pressure had stabilized, his fever was down, and he was beginning to wake up. Even the reddened area on his toes was beginning to recede. I stood there taking it all in, feeling triumphant, even heroic, claiming a lot of the credit. Frances came over to see how I was doing and I told her I thought we could probably start weaning down the settings on the ventila-tor and how I planned to get my patient up in the chair the next day.

"That's thinking like a nurse," she said.

"How does a nurse think?"

"Like the way you considered all the aspects of the situation and set goals, planned ahead. How you supported the family, explained everything to them. That kind of thing."

MY FIRST YEAR working in the ICU with Laura's Line was un-forgettable. I learned so much, and made wonderful friends. It was also the year my mother died after so many years of being so ill and the year in which I got married to Ivan, a South African man I'd met during my trip to Israel. He came to live with me in Toronto, we bought a house, and together made it a home. It was a surprising year. As I worked through the fresh grief over my mother's death and the residual grief over my father's, I found tremendous gratification at work and in my friendships with my colleagues, and enormous happiness in my private life. Unexpectedly, joyfulness overtook me. So, that year, the juxta-position of mourning and celebration made perfect sense to me. I had always known that sadness and happiness could coexist. And along with all of that, there was so much fun! Laura's Line made sure of that. No holiday, milestone, or birthday ever went uncele-brated. After work or on days off, we'd get together. Once, at a late-night karaoke bar, I got up on stage and belted out a mean version of "Hit Me With Your Best Shot," then Justine did her raunchy rendition of "Love Shack," which brought the house down. (Also memorable was the cake with green icing on St. Patrick's Day and the chocolate bars Laura brought in on Halloween that were shaped like skeletons and sarcophagi. And Justine was the first person I had ever heard use the word *party* as a verb.) We got about an hour or two of sleep those nights, even when we had to work the next morning. We were tired but we knew we could get through anything together. They were colleagues, soon became friends, and will always be my sisters.

7

HOCKEY MOM, RN

Many decisions in my life have been fraught with ambivalence and anxiety. But when it came time to ask my true love to marry me, I plucked up the courage. Luckily, he had no such hesitations.

"Yes, of course" was Ivan's immediate answer.

Eighteen years of marriage have been pretty good, mostly wonderful, in fact. Even during the first few years when Ivan, originally from South Africa, had to leave his thriving business and close family in Israel, the country he loves most, uproot himself, and join me in Canada, he never once complained or expressed any doubts about his choice. And over the years when inevitable misunderstandings and conflicts have arisen between us, he remains steadfast. "You make the decision to love someone and that's it. You don't stop" is how he puts it. And any doubts *I* might have had were completely banished one romantic evening about twelve years ago as we took a leisurely stroll in our new neighbourhood. I was nine months pregnant with our first child and I had a feeling it would be the last of such serene moments. Since Ivan was still fairly new to Canadian ways at that time, I felt it my duty to inform him about an essential requirement for our new citizen-to-be. "You know," I said as we strolled hand in hand. "If it's a boy, you will have to get up very early in the morning and take him to hockey practice."

Without missing a beat he answered, "And if it's a girl, I'll get up early and take her, too."

I don't think he knew how his comment made me love him more, if that was possible, and even more, since.

AT WORK THE OTHER DAY, I shared a laugh with the other nurses. It was right before starting our shift and we were gathered at the nursing station, checking our patient assignments. A few of us were chatting about our kids. "Can you believe it?" I asked them. "Me. A hockey mom!"

Because of our two hockey-playing sons, I have learned about hat tricks, drop passes, and one-timers. I have even begun to understand breakouts, offsides, and penalty kills. I am intimately familiar with the exact location of every hockey arena in Toronto. Yes, I have become a bona fide, albeit at times reluctant, hockey mom. But the nurses had reason to laugh because many of them still recall how I faced the prospect of motherhood: with a mix of excitement and dread, anticipation and fear. They tried hard to encourage me during my pregnancy.

About labour, Casey offered scary, yet reassuring, advice. "It feels like there's a train blasting through you and all you can do is hold on for dear life and pray you don't split in two. But you'll get through it."

I called George at home. He was on parental leave with his second child and had given me helpful information about epidurals during labour and now I had questions I wanted to ask him about episiotomies, but in the midst of our discussion he broke off: "Gotta go. There's diarrhea streaming out of Amelia's diaper."

Noreen noticed me reading a novel during my break. "Enjoy it now," she said grimly, "there'll be no time to read once the baby comes." I could have cried. I knew that everything was about to change and the problem was, I loved things just the way they were.

But then I thought about so many nurses I had known who struggled with infertility problems and how they longed for a baby. For
example, I knew just how badly Jenna yearned for one once when
I covered for her so she could take a break and happened to come
across her hopeful list jotted on the back of a lab report. "Corey,
Colin, Cathleen, Candice." I just knew they were potential baby
names. For Ivan and me, everything was going smoothly. Perhaps
it was time to be grateful.

Louise, a nurse I had worked with for a few years but whom I
didn't know very well at the time, came over to me on my last day
of work before my maternity leave to wish me well. I'd always
admired how she looked so young that her three grown-up kids
were often mistaken for her siblings. Louise's simple words of
advice have stayed with me over the years. "Enjoy it," she said with
a reassuring smile. "Have fun. Your kids will be happy if they see
you happy."

Of course. Is anything sadder than a sad mother?

I was determined above all else to be a fun, upbeat mother, but
nothing woke me up more to the reality of motherhood than a
moment upon returning to my hospital room a few hours after the
delivery of our healthy son. Ivan had gone home and the baby –
we named him Harry after my father – was asleep in a plastic
bassinet beside my bed. *I'll go have a shower*, I thought, *and
freshen up a bit after that little ordeal.* I donned my bathrobe and
gathered soap and shampoo.

Snap! Like a dog on a retractable leash, I was yanked back. I
couldn't do whatever, whenever I wanted any more! I was tied
forever to this new "patient" – a baby. He was mine, but he was a
stranger, and I didn't even know if I liked him yet! My old life was
over! I was now a *mother*. That word had always filled me with
apprehension. Luckily, a few hours later, Laura's Line arrived,
laden with gifts for the baby, treats and goodies for me. Frances
had knitted a tiny blue sweater and bonnet for the baby and she
showed me how to bathe him and soothe him when he wailed.
Nicky and I hugged each other and cried. Justine was busy flirting
with the obstetrics resident while Tracy cracked open a bottle of
champagne. Laura stood holding the baby at the window because

she detected neonatal jaundice due to a delayed clearance of bilirubin. It was common in newborns and direct sunlight was the treatment for it. It was wonderful having them there. I loved their company and they brought me back to myself. They reminded me that I was one of them – a nurse – capable, confident, and knowledgeable. I can handle this, I told myself, and I rose to the challenge.

SINCE I'VE ALWAYS BEEN a heavy sleeper, I worried that I might not hear the baby crying. But I recalled what a sales representative had told us about a new cardiac monitor as he demonstrated its many features. When he sounded the alarm, we were concerned. Its faint, tinkling sound seemed far too *unalarming*. "No worries. You'll hear it," he reassured us and then explained, "Scientists have isolated an acoustic 'sweet spot.' There's a specific quality in the cries of newborn babies that irritates the brain and we've put that technology into our equipment." Maybe it was like that for me because whenever Harry cried, I heard him and I got up and went. It was the most straightforward, unequivocal response of my life even in those moments when I could also hear another baby crying, the one inside of me, welling up with its needs, crying for a mother, too. But I didn't allow those distractions to disturb me. I focused on my "patient," and did a thorough "nursing assessment," ruling out the usual suspects: hunger, fatigue, wet diaper, etc. *I know what an emergency is. I have handled many. This is not an emergency.*

It turned out that what helped me the most as a mother were the things I learned as a nurse.

Harry was only about a month old and late one evening, I peeked in on him. He was sleeping and I tiptoed out. Of course I utterly loved him by then. I closed the door behind me and burst into tears. I would never hear all the music in the world! I would never be able to read all the books or travel the globe like I'd wanted to! Even if I lived to be a hundred, it would not be enough. Life was bearing down on me. I was having a recurring dream of not getting to the airport in time or running behind a train, trying to catch up.

"My life is over," I wailed to Ivan, plunking myself down at the kitchen table.

"What's wrong?" He was at the sink, washing the dishes.

"You don't understand anything!" I launched into a diatribe about women's enslavement to biology, the history of women's oppression in a patriarchal society, and about the physiological and psychological effects of hormone disruptions.

He placed a cup of tea and a cookie on a plate in front of me.

In other, equally irrational moments, I bemoaned my miserable childhood and my crazy family, but Ivan had zero tolerance for wallowing, blaming, or self-pity. "You can't keep using your family as an excuse. It's time to get over it," he said with a *click, click* of the TV remote control.

It seemed there was this mantle of maturity I was expected to wear as a mother. Clearly, the statute of limitations of being angry at my parents and holding them responsible for my problems was over. It was time to grow up. No, I didn't have parents, grand-parents, or siblings to rely on, but I had wonderful friends and something else – my own private twenty-four-hour hotline. At any time of day or night, I could call a colleague at work and receive practical advice. I learned about colic, teething, toilet training, and ear infections from my ICU family. I turned to them not only because many were mothers and fathers themselves, but because they were scientifically minded, well-read professionals who knew what they were talking about.

Still, I often felt lonely at home with my baby. Had there been online chat groups in cyberspace with other mothers back then, I might have done that, but it wasn't "parenting" I wanted to speak to them about. It was art, music, literature, and nursing. I wanted to find a way to stay connected to the outside world and at the same time, to the inside one, in between my baby and me.

ONE AFTERNOON, I was sitting in a rocking chair feeding Harry when I got a call from Dr. Darryl Price, who was a staff physician from the ICU. I was very fond of him and had always admired the exceptionally kind way he talked to patients and their families. He was calling to invite me to sit on a panel of critical care experts at a symposium to discuss the topic "When Medical Treatment Is Deemed Futile." I looked down at my pink terrycloth slippers and flannel nightgown, damp from leaking milk. The last time I'd seen him, I'd been wearing scrubs and a lab coat and he was explaining to me his research on the cellular inflammatory processes in septic shock.

"Futile?" I gazed down at my baby's milk-drunk face, the very antithesis of futility. "I can't talk about *that*, Darryl. Nurses don't believe in it. It's not a word nurses ever use."

"I'm referring to situations when there is no benefit in continuing treatment. When the decision is made to withdraw life support."

"I know what the *word* means . . . well, let me think about it. I'll get back to you."

He paused for a few seconds. "Was that enough time?"

I laughed, "Okay, I'll do it."

"I knew you'd come around," he chuckled.

Big mistake.

LATER THAT DAY while Harry was napping, I sat at my desk to make notes for my speech. Yes, I had cared for many patients who had no chance of survival and a number who had died. In so many cases, we had pressed on, performing more and more procedures, tests, and treatments, even when no member of the team truly believed there was any chance of benefit, often at the insistence of family members who wanted "everything done." Yet, in other similar situations, different choices were made. Whatever the decisions, what always troubled me the most was that we rarely knew directly from patients themselves what their wishes were. Even with those who had written "advance directives" or had appointed individuals as their decision-makers, when the time came, we were often uncertain how to proceed. It was never a clear-cut or easy decision.

Where did I stand in all of this? As a nurse, I knew exactly where I "stood": at the very nexus between the patient and the family, right in the space between the patient and the rest of the team. As nurses we are closest to the patient, both physically and metaphysically and thus, we are in the ideal position to see all sides. Yet, it is also that very proximal position and intimate role that makes us the most conflicted and distressed as we witness our patients' suffering on a daily and nightly basis.

I managed to prepare a speech and then turned to a more mundane challenge: What to wear to such a prestigious occasion? Since I swore I wouldn't buy new clothes until I'd lost my pregnancy weight, I managed to squeeze into an old plaid skirt and a black jacket over a blouse that was far too tight. It pulled across my chest and under my arms.

The first speaker was a physician who talked about the high mortality rates in the ICU and the futility of offering treatment that has no benefit to patients. The second speaker was an economist who spoke about the rising cost of health-care technology and the imperative to utilize precious health-care dollars judiciously. The third speaker was a lawyer who spoke so far above my head – and I was so anxious about my own speech – that I couldn't follow what he was saying. Then it was my turn. I glanced longingly at the exit door and slowly mounted the stairs to the podium. I looked out at the crowd. I had no Power Point presentation and no research to report, nor statistics to recite, but surely all my years of experience counted for something? I moved closer and took a huge breath. There was a screech and a squeal. *Oh, too close to the mike. Step back.* "Futility," I cleared my throat. "Futility is . . ." I looked down at the notes I had prepared and found them useless. I set them aside. "Futility is a concept that is not part of nursing's philosophy. It is not in most nurses' lexicons. I cannot imagine a situation where offering nursing care would be futile. I have never felt that anything I did as a nurse was futile. That's the beauty of nursing. We don't have dilemmas about futility, though we do have other dilemmas, I can assure you." *Laugh, laugh, laugh,* from the audience, which emboldened me to continue and tell them about the many times when I put aside my tasks and preoccupation with numbers and simply sat down and listened to patients and their families and tried to share the burden of their suffering. I described some of the many occasions when nurses believed that "comfort

measures" – simple human touch and caring – were more important than medical intervention. "Of course, we are saddened when
a patient dies, but for us it is not the defeat or failure it seems to
be for doctors," I acknowledged.

"In conclusion, I wish to quote one of my ICU mentors and
teacher Dr. Imré Sandor, who always says that 'while there may be
times when we may decide to withdraw *treatment*, we never withdraw *care*.' Thank you very much." I stepped down. My head was
pounding, I was dripping with sweat, my breasts were engorged,
and I was flushed with embarrassment at my remarks, so hokey,
sentimental, and simplistic. I'd been reading too many *Tales of
Thomas the Tank Engine* and not enough back issues of *Critical
Care Nursing*!

"I would like to take exception to two points raised by speaker
number four," someone said. *Yikes, that would be . . . me! What
would the Teletubbies do in this situation?* I can't recall the objec-
tions, but I answered as best I could. I was way out of my depth.
My mind had gone to mush. Futility! What was futile here was my
attempt to juggle everything – being a nurse, a mother, a wife, and
a homemaker all at the same time. I couldn't do it.

TOWARD THE END of my eight-month maternity leave, in the last
few weeks before returning to work, I joined a fitness centre.
They had a babysitting service and I intended to use those precious two hours to myself to exercise, but all too often, I put
them to a different use. On the sign-in sheet where you had to
indicate where you would be in case your baby needed you,
where the other mothers wrote, "Treadmill" or "Running
Track," I pencilled in "Cafeteria." I went there not to eat and
drink, but to read and think.

One day sitting there I looked up from my book as a tall, strik-
ing woman swept in. She wore a long black coat, a black velvet
hat, and bright red scarf. She carried herself regally and even the
way she plucked a few coins from her purse with long, manicured
fingers to pay for a bottle of water looked elegant. She smiled at
the cashier, as if her payment was a tip. I suddenly became aware

of my baggy sweatpants, T-shirt, and running shoes. For some reason, she caught sight of me and strode over, sipping her Perrier through a straw. "Hi, I'm Daphne Marcus. What are you reading?" She extended her hand. I had noticed her before in an exercise class, always in the front, facing the mirror, toes turned out and arms raised in a manner more suited to ballet than aerobics.

I introduced myself and showed her my book. It was *Angela's Ashes*. She gave a slight, involuntary shudder. "Oh, I can't read that. Such things make me weep."

Weep? "No, it didn't make me weep," I said. It wasn't just about sad, squalid circumstances, it was about overcoming those circumstances.

"By any chance are you a writer?" She pointed to the notebook on the table beside me.

"No, well, yes. I do write, but I haven't published anything." She said she was a poet and asked if I would like to write with her and critique each other's work. I jumped up. "There's just this one thing . . ."

"What? If it's your dream, don't let any obstacles get in your way."

"I have a baby. In fact I have to pick him up from the baby-sitting room right now. I'm late." But before I ran off, she pulled out her diary and we set a date. I didn't have to pull out mine because I knew it was empty.

WE MET at a downtown café called Mocha Mocha. Harry napped co-operatively in his car seat on a chair beside me. (Daphne had a teenaged son but offered me a useful tip she recalled from her own baby days. If I allowed my left breast to fill up all morning, by the time I got to the writing table in the afternoon, I could tuck the baby in place and my right hand would be free to write my heart out.) We ordered cappuccino and discussed Virginia Woolf and Jane Austen, but as soon as Harry woke up I was able only to add a comment here or there because I was also busy chasing down a squeaky plastic porcupine across the room where he kept flinging it. Just then, four mothers walked in, each pushing a stroller. They took up places around a large oval table and settled in to eat lunch and lift their shirts to feed their babies. They commiserated about how little sleep they were getting and debated the relative eco-qualities of disposable versus cloth diapers. *That table is where I should be. Here I am trying to be a writer . . . Why can't I be satisfied just being a mother?* I watched Daphne fill pages with a fountain pen, applying ink with dashes and flourishes, the way a painter would splash colour and texture all over a canvas.

"I'm stuck," I told her, capping my pen. "I don't have anything to write about."

She looked up. "Writer's block is indulgence. It's about procrastination and fear. If you want to write, you have to write in every mood, even if it's difficult."

I shook my head. "I can't do it."

"Write something that will delight me," Daphne advised.

"I can't think of anything."

"Write about your sex life in Israel," she suggested, "or your New York adventures, like those Fifth Avenue shopping sprees or the all-night parties with those celebrities on the Upper West Side."

I uncapped my pen, put it to the paper, and have done so every single day since then, almost twelve years ago. Once a week, Daphne and I met in a Starbucks or at the Moonbeam Café, the Golden Griddle, or jazz clubs where we would sip wine and improvise in our own way. We chose places where the servers were either indifferent or else ignored us and we always left a decent tip. After we ate, always sooner than I felt ready, Daphne set aside her food, dabbed at her lips with a serviette, and reapplied her lipstick: these were the signals that it was time to get to work.

Daphne spun out poems about beauty and romantic love. One was about an erotic relationship between a cello, a saxophone, and a piano. Some were even about secret, forbidden love and passionate affairs with lovers' limbs intertwined like pretzels. Daphne rarely faltered, but when she did she had only to pull out a handful of the paint chips she carried with her and the names of colours such as Blue Reef, Colonial Red, or Peony Blush would be enough to stoke her imagination.

I wrote too, but not nearly as prodigiously. If I filled ten note-books during our time together, Daphne must have filled one hundred. We had many lovely times together and the only note of discord between us was when I wrote *certain* stories.

"Scary," she would say, covering her ears. "It's too depressing," she said about my hospital stories. I apologized and began to avoid subjects that might disturb her. But those other stories continued to haunt me. I was beginning to realize that there were some things only nurses knew and shared among themselves. Nurses had lots of stories that had never been told publicly before, only privately, in hallways or stairwells, outside elevators, in whispers and in secret. I began to write them on my own at home, away from Daphne.

"Do you have any idea what I do, sitting at my desk?" I asked Ivan one day. He was making a salad and I was watching him rinse the lettuce. *It is hard living with a non-artist*, I thought. *He doesn't understand me. Maybe I should leave him? I need to go off some-where by myself!*

"You think. You write."

I guess I'll stay.

TWO AND A HALF YEARS LATER, in 1997, I became a mother for the second time with the birth of Max. It was a much easier transition this time, though credit is also due to Barney, the purple TV dinosaur who babysat Harry during the first few weeks. During that happy time, I received upsetting news in the form of a letter from the hospital. It was a layoff notice. I became one of hundreds of nurses whose jobs were cut all across the Province of Ontario in a new mandate called "health-care restructuring." I was one of the lucky ones offered the option of "re-deployment" (again, the military terminology) to a "relief pool." What a misnomer that was! There was no relief to be had and the only thing remotely aquatic about it was that you had to sink or swim. I would no longer be a critical care nurse or belong to a team. I would be a generic worker in a large corporation, expected to fill in wherever "labour units" were short. Stunned, I considered my options.

Meanwhile, as hospitals madly scrambled to care for patients, administrators once again came to the obvious realization that the so-called *surplus* of nurses was, in fact, quite the opposite – a *shortage* of nurses. I reapplied to my old job in the ICU and was able to return, this time in a part-time position. Going part-time was my choice back then, but many nurses didn't have that luxury and had to patch together a number of jobs in various hospitals in order to bring in a full-time salary to support their families, now as casual workers, without benefits.

Returning to work after a second long maternity leave, three years later, it didn't take me long to regain my groove. And during that time, without fail, every week, Daphne and I continued to meet. Until one day, after six years of writing together, I realized the time had come to break away from her. There were stories I wanted to tell but felt I couldn't in her presence for fear of upsetting her. By bowing out, I was protecting both of us, she from hearing my disturbing stories and myself from frustration at having to squelch, or at best, sugarcoat them. Daphne was angry when I ended our partnership that for such a long time had been so productive for both of us. In time, I think she forgave me. At any rate, she went on to publish two books of poetry, and years later, a third. But neither of us could have known or imagined in those days that within only a few years Daphne would be diagnosed with an illness herself and be forced to enter the world of the hospital. But back then, if she preferred not to think about such unpleasantness, who could blame her?

8

YOUR MOTHER, YOUR FATHER

I t takes a nurse to teach a nurse. There have been many teachers along the way for me and now I teach others. It's relatively easy to show someone how to insert a naso-gastric tube to decompress a patient's stomach. Adjusting the ventilator to improve a patient's arterial blood gases is a more complex skill. It's even more complicated to teach someone how to attend to the multitude of details required to manage a patient in multi-system organ failure. But I still haven't figured out how to teach another nurse to manage the emotions this work can evoke. I know many experienced nurses who still struggle with this challenge. How do you care, but not so much that it hurts? How do you make your care patient-centred, yet still keep your personal boundaries intact? There are huge emotional risks in caring for critically ill people. This work can break your heart.

I began to understand something about these boundaries one night a few years ago during a hockey game. It was the Stanley Cup playoffs, in a match between the Toronto Maple Leafs and the Detroit Red Wings. A Detroit player slammed into Maple Leafs goalie Curtis "Cujo" Joseph, who got angry and hit back.

Well, the gloves came off and the punches started flying. The refer-
ees had to pry the players apart to end the brawl. Then, when they
must have assumed the camera was off, Cujo lifted his goalie mask
(that depicted a ferocious beast) and mouthed to his rival, "You
okay?" The opponent nodded and pointed with his chin, "You?"
Seeing that tender, sincere moment helped me understand something about nursing, the place to which for me, all roads lead. Not
that I ever saw myself as an adversary with any of my patients – not
at all – but it is so easy to imagine that the gap between them, the
sick ones, and us, the healthy ones, is much vaster than it is.
Sometimes I took off my mask, too, and went over to the other side.
But in my need for intimacy and my desire to rescue others, I often
took on patients' emotions in ways that helped neither of us.

For many years, I took off my mask and crossed over frequently
and sloppily. Perhaps it was how I learned as a child to care for my
mother by sharing her sadness. I showed her my love by feeling her
pain. Growing up, my personal boundaries were always uncertain.
So often, my own emotions blended and mixed with whatever
others around me were experiencing. When I became a nurse, I continued on in that style of caring, even though it made things worse
for me and sometimes for my patients, too. They needed to feel that
I was steady and in control, but I couldn't always offer them that
security. I caught their emotions as if they were contagious.
Sometimes, merely being in the presence of a patient, family
member, or even another nurse, who was flustered, anxious, or
angry would affect me, and I would respond in tandem. Patients
may even have felt they had to take care of *me*. Too often, I was a
gushing, emoting heart that rendered me less effective as a nurse.
Nurses are supposed to keep their emotions under control, but it's
been a struggle for me.

WHEN I THINK OF Mr. Salvatore, I think of his daughter, Yvette.
Mr. Salvatore was a seventy-two-year-old with esophageal cancer
who developed abscesses throughout his abdomen. The doctors
were hopeful that they could drain them and that he would then

be well enough to undergo surgery to remove the cancer. In the meantime, he went into respiratory failure and had to be admitted to the ICU. Every day Yvette stayed at his side. She kept her eyes locked on me the whole time, watching every move I made. When I went to suction his lungs, she leaped out of her chair. "Should I panic?" she asked, searching my face for clues as to how she should react.

"No need to panic," I said extra calmly and slowly. "Your dad is doing just fine."

"Look, Daddy, your nurse is smiling. She wouldn't smile if things weren't looking good."

Yvette asked me if she could go home for a little rest. I knew she wanted my reassurance that nothing bad would happen while she was away from her father's side. With her eyes she implored me, *I need to rest, shower, see my kids. Please grant me permission to do so.* I wanted to tell her to go home and take care of herself but I didn't dare. If something did happen while she was gone, she would never forgive me. She left briefly only for a coffee and a phone call. "Take good care of him while I'm gone," she pleaded, throwing kisses at her father as she left. "He's special. He's my dad."

Later that afternoon, when Mr. Salvatore's heart suddenly went into an erratic rhythm, Yvette was right there at his side. When the alarm sounded, she grabbed my arm. "I'm panicking!" she shouted. I tried to calm her down and deal with the emergency at the same time. The doctor came in and ordered an intravenous beta-blocker to slow the heart rate. Shortly after I gave it, Mr. Salvatore's cardiac problem was resolved, but no amount of reassurance I offered eased his daughter's anxiety. Later that day, Mr. Salvatore had to be transported to another part of the hospital for the radiologist to drain the abscesses in his belly.

"Is *this* reason to panic?" Yvette asked, clasping my hand. In answer, I put one arm around her and pushed the bed along with my other hand as we made our way down the hall to the procedure room. There, the radiologist met with her and told her that if the "collections" turned out not to be fluid-filled then he wouldn't be able to drain them. "In that case, I can't do anything," he said as the technician spread out a green sterile drape over the patient's abdomen in preparation for the procedure.

"What does that mean?" she asked him. "Does that mean it's serious?"

"It means I can't drain it," the doctor said without further elaboration. Draining abscesses under fluoroscopy was his specialty, but for whatever reason he didn't explain that if there wasn't fluid to be drained, then it was probably a solid mass, such as a tumour, and in this case, likely malignant. But Yvette sensed the ominous implication. "Are you saying it would be bad?" The radiologist was preoccupied, already in the midst of the procedure, so she turned back to me, but I was busy giving her father sedation and assisting the doctor with the procedure. Out of the corner of my eye, I saw her terror-stricken face, her tiny, rigid body that looked like it might snap in two. She held on to her pale forehead. "I'm panicking," she said in a tremulous voice. I looked around the room for a chair and luckily, just then, the technician caught her as she keeled over. Full-blown panic had finally done her in, but at least it allowed me to now focus my attention on taking care of her father. I exhaled. I hadn't realized how shallow my breathing had become, how tight my chest was, how jittery I felt. I had caught a bad case of her panic.

I'VE WORKED WITH Noreen for the past ten years or so. She has a tough, abrasive personality and often has a sour look of disapproval on her face, but I have learned to ignore it because she's really very kind-hearted and an excellent nurse. Noreen is someone who always seems to have her emotions under control, even the day she took care of a patient whose family pushed her to the limit.

Loud and clear we all heard a terrible drama playing out in the corner room. A young man had been brought to the ICU in fulminant liver failure, a life-threatening consequence from the anabolic steroids he'd been taking for bodybuilding. The waiting room was jampacked with visitors, all wanting to see him, so many that they spilled out into the hall.

"Are all those people *family*?" someone asked Noreen, who was his nurse that day. "There are cans of Coke and bags of potato chips everywhere and they reek of cigarettes and alcohol. You should inform them that only two visitors at a time are allowed and they have to call in first."

"To me, family is whoever they say they are," Noreen said in her matter-of-fact manner. "As far as I'm concerned, they can come in whenever they want. The kid is going to die."

On one side of the bed, a slim teenaged girl wearing a doo rag and tattered jeans was doubled over, sobbing. On the other side, sat an older woman wearing a dress that draped her body like a tent. "That's the girlfriend and that's the mother," Noreen whispered. I had heard vicious screaming going on and had come over to give Noreen a hand, but she didn't seem to need my help.

"You just want a piece of him," the mother shouted at the girl, "you fuckin' whore!"

Noreen stood at the foot of the bed, a bit closer to the girlfriend. "Now, now," she clucked. "Keasha loves him, too."

"Yeah, right," the mother snarled. "Jerome has lots of chicks and this here bitch is only one of 'em. He's my boy. I want her the hell out of here." She lunged across the bed to take a swing at Keasha, but Noreen grabbed her arm and stopped her in time. "You better control yourself, or you'll have to leave." She pulled up a chair for Keasha, who smiled sweetly but then retaliated in an equally nasty manner. "I hate you," she screamed at the mother, "and Jerome hates you, too. He told me so."

"That's enough," Noreen snapped, but then softened. "Easy does it, sweetie. Take a deep breath. Think before you speak."

"Alls I wanted to do was wipe his forehead, but *she*," Keasha glared across the bed at the mother, "slapped my hand." She turned to the safety of Noreen. "Something like this has never happened to me before." She fell onto Noreen and cried into her shoulder. "I never had a sick boyfriend."

"Of course not, you're still a baby," Noreen put her arm around her, and held her close, comforting her the way a mother would her child. "You're so young to have to go through this."

"It's not her going through this, it's Jerome," the mother said, pointing at her son, who was completely unconscious and unaware of the storm taking place, literally, over his body. "A piece of work like her'll get herself another boyfriend, but I'll never get myself another son." She caressed his arm.

"Jerome's going to make it," Keasha said. "You've given up on him."

"You're nothing but a fuckin' ho!" shouted the mother, gripping the side rails of the bed and hauling herself to her feet. "You have no right to even be here."

"Yes, I do, you bitch!" The girlfriend lunged at her neck, but Noreen held her back. "We're getting married," she held up her hand to reveal a ring with a blue stone in it. "Jerome loves me. He told me how you abused him and screwed up his life."

Noreen stared at them over the top of her bifocals. "Both of you are disturbing my patient. Now, you better show respect for Jerome. He's the focus here. Get a grip or get out!"

"You can't get rid of me. I'm his mother." She settled back down into the chair and crossed her arms across her chest.

The war continued all day. It was ugly and unrelenting, but it didn't flap Noreen in the least. She focused on caring for her patient in her usual calm, methodical manner and on supporting all members of the family as best she could. Meanwhile, Jerome's condition was deteriorating. He began to vomit blood and suddenly had a seizure that deepened his coma. His blood pressure was dropping and the Ph, oxygen, carbon dioxide, and bicarbonate levels in his arterial blood gases began to reach dangerously abnormal amounts, indicating that he was near death.

"Jerome is dying," the liver specialists told them. "There is nothing more we can do. His liver has been damaged beyond repair and unfortunately he is too sick to be listed for a transplant. We are very sorry." Then they left.

This news made the mother and girlfriend even more violent. They lunged at each other. The girl scratched the mother's face and neck. The mother yanked the girl's hair. Noreen sprang into action. "That's it! Get out, the two of you! Take it outside. I'm calling security." But before they could arrive, the mother stomped out of the ICU and Keasha fled to the waiting room. Noreen looked at me with the same exasperated expression I had seen on her face at the behaviour of her own teenaged kids. Otherwise, as far as I could tell, she remained unperturbed by the chaos swirling around her, steadfast in the face of the impending, inevitable tragedy. She was a calm centre around which the two of them could safely rage.

The problem was, you weren't supposed to speak like this to patients. The scripts we had been taught as students, the stock phrases and prescribed responses we were supposed to offer, such as "you seem angry," "what are your concerns?" or "what is this situation like for you?" were inadequate for many of the extreme situations we encountered in the ICU. Noreen spoke to this family in the same way I'd heard her speak to her own kids when they misbehaved. She tried to bring them into line. She scolded them. She took a stand and called them on their bad behaviour. She used her own pragmatic personality and no-nonsense, straight-talking manner to nurse this family, and it seemed the perfect way to handle the situation.

Later that day, Jerome had a cardiac arrest and no further resuscitation efforts were attempted. His mother and his girlfriend had no more energy to expend on their anger, as they were forced to expend it on their grief. Noreen removed all of the tubes, IVs, machines, and pieces of equipment attached to Jerome and then she bathed his body thoroughly and put fresh sheets on the bed. Then she brought his mother and girlfriend back into the room, along with other members of the family, and allowed them to be with his body for as long as they wished. Noreen stayed strong and silent amidst the room full of mourners who were wailing and pulling at their hair and clothing in their anguish. Other nurses came over to offer their support, as well, but I had my patient to get back to and my own work to do. I got busy and didn't think any more about them.

At the end of the shift, I found Noreen sitting on the bench in the locker room, sobbing uncontrollably. She apologized for her emotions. "I guess I got too involved." She wiped her face and stood up. "I don't know what happened. I usually never let myself go there." I waited while she slowly put on her coat. We were planning to meet

up with a few other nurses for drinks, but Noreen bowed out. She
said she was tired and was going home instead.

YES, I'LL ADMIT IT: certain patients still crank me up, especially the
angry, distrustful ones or the combative, hostile ones. I feel more
comfortable around patients who are sad or depressed, perhaps
because those emotions are more familiar to me. Expressions of
emotion from the nurse mean a lot to families. When I cry with
them, they appreciate that I share their grief. Sometimes it seems
to matter more to families how sympathetic I am than how skilled
I am. When they see how hard it is for us, too, somehow it light-
ens their burden.

Patients expect nurses, and nurses expect themselves, to make
every effort to see, feel, and understand a patient's experiences. But
all too often, when I did that, I became overwhelmed with
someone else's sorrows. I lost myself. I came to realize that I wasn't
going to be able to stay in this profession if I didn't change my
ways. I had to learn how to safely enter a patient's world and still
keep mine intact.

We once had a social worker who came up with the idea that
the nurses should make more of an effort to attend patients'
memorial services, to stay in touch with grieving families, send
them sympathy cards, and even pay them visits in their homes to
help them find "closure." I wasn't the only nurse who felt uneasy
with this plan.

"Don't include me in on that," one nurse told her sharply.
"Some of us need to make a separation. Most of us do."

The social worker looked even more dismayed when I expressed
my opinion that some families might not wish to have any
reminders of the ICU if their loved one had died there. She seemed
to consider anything less than a full, emotional demonstration,
replete with weeping and moaning, to be cold and callous. She
would sit with families and commiserate with them about every
setback. She told them about her own problems. She had such
demonstrably personal reactions to patients, especially select ones
who suffered from diseases her own friends and family members

had lived through, such as HIV and psychiatric illnesses. But who was I to judge? I had my own weaknesses. I always broke down when children came into the ICU to say goodbye to grandparents, or even parents. When one little boy said to his mom, "It doesn't look like Daddy on the outside, but it's still Daddy on the inside, isn't it?" well, I lost it altogether. Once, when I found a clipboard with the one word *perché?* which I knew was "why?" in Italian, scribbled by a dying old man, I burst into tears.

For a time I thought that perhaps the way to counterbalance my emotional nature would be to hold myself back. *What would happen*, I asked myself, *if I didn't try to connect personally with each and every patient and family?* I would give correct, safe care, of course, but maintain a dispassionate stance and keep my guard up. I would not take off my mask and go over to the other side. After all, didn't Laura always say you didn't have to get to know your patient in order to give good care? What about Frances, who always gave so much of herself but never let her emotions get out of control? "When you come to work," she told me on many occasions, "leave yourself at the door." She believed it was her function to ensure her patient's well-being. "I treat all my patients as if they're members of my family," she explained to me. But still, how did she do it, I wondered?

Justine was a nurse who willingly took on emotional risks, but eventually it got the better of her, and I think it was the reason she ended up leaving the ICU. She once was furious at a family that never visited their grandmother, yet kept calling to insist that "everything be done" to resuscitate her. Justine hung up the phone on them and returned to her patient. She looked down at the frail old woman, pushed the machines aside, parted the tubes and lines with her hands, crawled right into the bed and lay down beside her. I can still see that lady's soft white hair and Justine cradling her in her strong arms and rocking her like a baby.

My problem was that I got into too many patients' beds! I felt their despair. I worried along with the family. At times, I even took their pain home with me. I decided to make that conscious effort to hold back, not let myself feel too much. I kept focused on numbers and facts and didn't make myself as readily available for patients to tell me their stories. I lasted about a week. I had made such a complete disconnect from feelings that my actions began to feel empty and meaningless. Caring for patients became drudgery and every task a chore. Without emotions to fuel me there was only logic and reasoning to figure out what was needed and my sense of duty to carry it through. I couldn't find a balance between my emotional nature and the rational thinking required to be a nurse. There had to be an alternative to losing myself or else keeping strictly within the confines of my nursing role, as if it were part of my uniform. I knew that only by bringing those two sides together could I be the nurse I wanted to be.

Many nurses struggle with the emotional stress of our work, yet rarely talk about it. I have long suspected that burn-out and the disproportionately high rates of smoking, drinking, substance abuse, and depression among nurses, and the high numbers of sick days that nurses are known to experience aren't entirely due to the physical demands of our work, yet there are plenty of those. But I have always recovered from the sore backs caused by lifting heavy patients and the headaches after a stretch of night shifts. I've even had needlestick injuries that caused me worry for weeks, but that fortunately didn't cause serious harm. Once, I was splashed in the face by spray from a ventilator accidentally disconnected from a patient with hepatitis C. Droplets of sputum melted in my eyes as I yelled, "Cover for me!" and ran out. Laura was there and she grabbed a bottle of sterile saline, clamped my eyelids open, and poured the whole bottle of fluid into my eyes, drenching me all over. I worried for weeks, but as it turned out, I didn't get infected, after all.

It seems that almost every nurse has a war story or two.

Casey recently reported an ailment that was serious, but in her telling, at least, fairly amusing. We were sitting at the nurses' station late one night when she launched into her latest drama. "I swear, I had the worst diarrhea of my life after taking care of that patient with *C. diff.*[*] This place is such a cesspool we should wash our hands *before* going to the bathroom. I was shitting myself, literally.

---

[*] *Clostridium difficile* is a bacterium that causes diarrhea.

There were no safe farts. I had only to hold the little specimen bottle over my butthole to give the doctor a sample, can you picture this?"

Unfortunately, I could, yet Casey felt it necessary to enact a pantomime with an empty Styrofoam cup before continuing on with her rant. "The manager called to challenge me about my sick time. The nerve of her to imply that I would take advantage of the system!"

It was lucky for her that Monica was not on that night, as she also would have taken her to task about her sick time. Monica was a nurse with keen ambitions and vowed when she was manager of an ICU, she would crack down on malingerers and abusers of the system. But how was she going to distinguish between those individuals (if there were such fraudulent claims) and all the legitimate complaints such as Casey's? Every one of us had to some degree or another experienced the real hazards of our work. We knew that most nurses' sick time was but a partial compensation for taking the brunt of only some of the very real risks of this work.

I SPENT MANY YEARS searching for my way of being a nurse. It's only been in recent years that I've learned how to take off my mask and not strip off my entire uniform along with it. Because if becoming a nurse has taught me one thing, it was that there are a lot more helpful things to offer a person than feel their pain. As a nurse there is so much you can *do* for people.

I took care of Evelyn McDermott many times during her long stay with us and got to know her and her family well. I'd always noticed how some families adorn patients' rooms with beautiful objects, messages, letters, signs, pictures, and photographs. Mrs. McDermott's three sons and her daughter, Carly, went beyond mere decoration. They transformed the entire room into a celebration of their mother. They covered the walls with photographs and a huge sign that announced: "Thank you to all of my caregivers." Through the stories the children told, and the ones revealed by the photographs, I got to know Evelyn McDermott as a woman and as their mother.

She was a single mom who'd raised her children on her own, a hockey mom, a master bridge teacher, superb baker, generous friend, and marathon runner – up until she got lung cancer. As a mother she had recognized and nurtured the talents and abilities of each of her children, especially the one son, a gifted athlete who became a professional baseball player.

"Too bad you didn't know my mom," her daughter, Carly, said. "I mean before she got sick."

"I am getting to know her," I said, "through you and your brothers."

Carly smiled. It was true. They were a lovely family and everyone enjoyed taking care of them. We cut them a lot more slack than most other families, letting them come and go as they pleased, even letting them participate in daily rounds and view their mother's X-rays and lab reports. One day, Carly went around the ICU and placed a small bar of Godiva chocolate beside each nurse's computer. On the label was a picture of a Florentine-style angel. There was something about this family's love for their mother that brought out the angelic in all of us who had the privilege of caring for them.

Around the clock, either Carly or one of her brothers was at their mother's side, spelling off the others so that everyone could get some rest. They became skilled at interpreting medical information and knew exactly what each test result meant and what each waveform on the monitor signified. A tiny improvement in the numbers made them rejoice. They sank back down again with each and every setback, big or small. They wanted to help with their mother's care and most nurses made that possible for them, but some had a harder time giving up control over the way things were done and handing over their responsibilities to the family.

When the time came to choose whether to opt for yet another surgery, the family did their homework. They went on the Internet and became thoroughly knowledgeable about the options. They deliberated for many days, weighing the pros and cons. It was a difficult decision because, as the surgeon explained, without this surgery she would die, but even with it, he admitted, she might die.

During rounds, the eldest son said to the staff doctor. "We want to ask you something."

"Sure, shoot," said the doctor cheerfully.

I looked at the son's face and knew what he was about to ask. No, please, not *that* question, I prayed silently. But I could see it coming and there was no way to stop it.

"What would *you* do if this were your mother?"

Your mother, your father. It's the most telling, the most provocative, potentially the most truth-extracting question of all. I watched the sharp, jutting angle of the doctor's Adam's apple sink deep into his neck. He swallowed hard and looked down at his shoes. What the family couldn't possibly know, but I knew, was that this doctor's own mother had died from breast cancer, just a few weeks ago. He was mourning the loss of his own mother at the same time as he was being called upon to show empathy for the possibility of this family's losing theirs. Of course he did not mention his private grief, nor reveal his own feelings in any way. "It's completely your decision," he said, putting the responsibility squarely back on their shoulders and launched once again into the various choices before them.

"We need our mother to be well," Carly implored him. "Help us make the right decision."

His eyes showed concern. He swallowed again. He didn't speak. I think he couldn't.

"She must get better. She's our mother," Carly offered by way of explanation for her "demanding behaviour." "Can you understand how we feel?"

He nodded and cleared his throat a few times, as if something was lodged there. He patted her gently on the arm and then moved to the next room, pushing along the portable computer that we use to display X-rays and lab reports during morning rounds.

The McDermott family chose to go ahead with the surgery and Evelyn improved rapidly, but became dependent on the ventilator for a long time afterward, now breathing through a tracheostomy – an opening in her neck. I was her nurse on the first day she was strong enough to take a few steps by herself. That day we also closed off her trach for a few minutes with a cork and that allowed her to finally speak. I was reminded once again how startlingly intimate and personal it is to hear a patient's voice for the first time. At first it was raspy and hoarse, but later in the day, when we corked her trach again, she conversed more freely, even cracking a few jokes. She gave me her prized secret recipe for her signature cake that oddly enough called for a can of 7-Up. Carly and I found a lot in common and exchanged e-mail addresses so we could keep in touch once her mother went home.

How false it would have felt to stay within the limitations of my strictly professional role with this family. How much I would have missed! I was responding to them as personally as I was professionally. I was their nurse, but I was also interacting with them like their friend. I couldn't help myself because I liked them and knew so well what it was like to be the daughter of a sick mother.

Later that day when I saw that Evelyn was tiring, but reluctant to rest and possibly disappoint Carly, I intervened. "Evelyn, you can close your eyes now and do your work while I do mine."

She looked relieved, but asked, "What's my work?"

"Breathing. Resting," I said.

Later, Carly wanted to bathe her mother and give her a back rub and I set up a basin, towels, and everything they would need for her to do so and gave them privacy. The nurses had even taught Carly how to suction her mother and clean her tracheostomy site and she did that, too. I wanted to caution Carly to slow down and pace herself. There was still a long haul ahead and plenty of time to do more, but she told me that her mother was not a burden. "I love taking care of her," she said. "I love her. I love her body. We'll take her home in any condition." Carly showed no signs of faltering. The more she did for her mother, the more she wanted to do. Every act was motivated by pure love and I was in awe of this mother and daughter, because to me that bond has always been a mystery. "Mom, you've just got to get better! I'm watching over you and I won't let anything bad happen," Carly promised. She covered her mother with a quilt she had made and sat beside her to watch a movie.

There was something else happening here and I knew it. Carly was the youngest, with three older brothers, just like me. She was the same age as me and had two young sons as I do. She loved the same books I did and also made quilts in her spare time, as I do. She did Sudoku puzzles to calm her mind; I did them too, for the same reason. She gave devoted, whole-hearted, loving care to her sick mother and I – well, there the similarities ended, but I enjoyed being in the presence of the two of them loving each other.

Complications set in. Evelyn spiked a high temperature. Infection developed and the surgeon came to take her back to the operating room. "She will die without this surgery," he said, handing a pen and consent form to Carly to sign. This time she had no hesitation. "I always told Mom that if you want to live, I will help to enhance your life in every way I can. If you decide you want to die, we accept that and we'll help ease your way out. So far, she keeps giving us the sign that she wants to fight."

Once again, Evelyn recovered. Day by day she improved. One afternoon, I spent time talking with Carly, her mother too weak to do much more than nod at us from time to time and hold Carly's hand. I put the radio close to her bed and she and her daughter sat there, listening to the baseball game and cheering for her son, Carly's brother's team. At the end of the day I got ready to leave and Carly came over to hug me. She told me that my strength that day had helped her to be strong. She whispered that she didn't want me to go, but said it genuinely, not as some families did to cast aspersion on other nurses. I said goodbye and when I looked back, I saw them sitting together, absorbed in the game.

Sometimes it is only the clock that frees me at the end of my shift; it allows me to put a limit, or a boundary, around my caring. Without it, I might not know to stop. I gave my report to the night nurse. I walked out the door and began to release all that I had seen and felt from my mind and from my body. I fell into my reliable ritual that liberates me from Planet ICU. I start by swinging my now-empty lunch bag as I call out goodbye to my friends. I trudge up the stairs to the locker room, always at a slower pace than when I started the shift and tripped down those same stairs long ago, that morning. I hang up my stethoscope and lab coat in my locker. Bundle up my dirty uniform and bang the locker door shut with my foot. Glance in the mirror over the sink as I sail past. Waiting for the elevator, I think about dinner, trying to decide if I will go through with the complicated mushroom risotto that I bought all the ingredients for (it has to be stirred and stirred over the heat until the moment it is served) or if I'm too impatient for that and will pop a frozen pizza in the oven. I push the revolving hospital door and inhale the city air as I step back out onto Planet Earth. By the time I'm on the subway, riding home, I have begun to re-acquaint myself with thoughts of my own family. By then I have put the McDermott family completely out of my mind. It's what I have to do.

So I was completely unprepared for what happened a few days later. I was on a day off and was at home reading the morning newspaper. I rarely read the sports section, but something there caught my eye. It was a half-page article with a photograph. The mother of a baseball player had died suddenly, unexpectedly at a Toronto hospital. She had been the team mother and mascot and the players had been rooting for her recovery. It was Evelyn McDermott. *How could it be? She was doing so well. What had I missed?* I seized the phone and called the ICU. I spoke with the nurse who had taken over from me that day. She told me about the arrest that occurred a few hours after I'd left. They'd worked on her until three o'clock in the morning. Everyone was there, the baseball star son arriving straight from his game.

"I'd never seen anything like it, Tilda. The family was right there and shouting at us the whole time. 'Do more compressions! Shock her again! Go up on the inotropes! Don't stop.' It was as if they were calling the code. When we finally stopped, she died immediately and we didn't even have to tell them. They knew. They knew in a way they wouldn't have if we'd kept them out. They had to see for them-selves that everything was being done and what everything being done looked like."

Then the doctor came on the phone, the one who had been there that day and all that night, too. He also felt unsettled about such an unexpected death. The autopsy report had not provided any concrete answers, only that there was nothing obvious we had missed. I hung up the phone and sat back. What did I feel? Two things: very sorry for their loss and genuinely proud of the care

I had given. I have come to accept that this is the emotional cost for the privilege of doing this work. The price is steep, but I am prepared to pay it. To me, it's worth it.

The funeral, the nurse had told me, was that very day. A few of the nurses were going, and they asked if I wanted to join them. "No thanks," I said. I rarely went to patients' funerals, wakes, shivas, or visitations, even though there were times I was tempted and this was surely one of them. So, what did I do? I stayed home and wrote it all down. It's my way of remembering, of honouring.

9

THE PROPER USE OF THE F-WORD

A s one of the few Jewish nurses where I work, I am often called upon to explain the religious rituals and laws that affect the care of our Jewish patients. The others realize I'm not an Orthodox Jew (*un*orthodox is more like it) but they still turn to me to answer their questions. I am usually out of my depth and have to run off to consult with an authoritative source, but the questions keep coming at me: What is the significance of the number eighteen? What is a bar mitzvah? Why, when a Jewish patient dies, is it necessary for someone to stay with the body at all times?* In turn, I have asked Muslims about the Koran, their prayers, and their halal foods, and Buddhists about their rituals and philosophy, as well as Christians, Catholics, Hindus, Zoroastrians, about theirs. Nowhere do religious beliefs come up more than in situations of life and death – especially death.

---

* The number eighteen has the numerical value of the word *life*. A bar mitzvah is a coming-of-age ceremony at the age of thirteen. A corpse is not allowed to be left alone in order that the soul, which is in a state of bewilderment, will be accompanied and safeguarded until the time of burial.

In our morning rounds in the ICU we often discuss the many ethical dilemmas that arise from our work. We usually discuss these matters as if they were strictly based on science and ethical principles, but often I think they come down to religion and values: what people believe and what they hold dear. And when that's the case, I've learned to back right off. If I do have an opinion, I keep it to myself. I have worked hard not to allow my personal values to affect the care I give my patients. Yet, other nurses find ways to use their religious beliefs in therapeutic ways.

Phoebe, for example, is a born-again Christian and one of a small, but growing, group of nurses who speak openly about their religious beliefs and allow them to pervade what they say and do as nurses. "If I say 'praise the Lord,' or 'God bless you,'" Phoebe said, "it opens a door for some people."

I have seen how a simple, well-placed comment like that from certain nurses did provide valuable opportunities for patients and families to find solace and communion. Many times I came upon Phoebe and other openly religious nurses praying with patients and families at the bedside. But some people maintain there's no place in nursing for this kind of religious ministering, that nursing should be non-denominational and unaffiliated in order to avoid bias, prejudice, and especially, coercion. Justine used to tease Phoebe about her religious fervour. Once, when Phoebe said, "The most important things in life are God, my family, and my job," Justine sidled up to her and poked her in the ribs, "Did you say *dog*?" She'd further deflate Phoebe's evangelical zeal by reminding her once again that she was one of the few people on the planet who didn't know who Elvis Presley was or tried to get a rise out of her with a comment like, "Come on, Phoebe, which is more important, how frequently couples pray together or have sex together?" which would make Phoebe blush and fall silent – until the next time.

Justine was raised a Catholic but the only "religion" she prac- tised was Compassion. She was guided by what she believed was the kindest course of action. One of the last patients she took care of in the ICU was Mr. Housden, an elderly man with Alzheimer's disease who came from a nursing home. He'd been found slumped over in his wheelchair, lips blue, and vital signs barely detectable. He was intubated and brought to the ICU. After a few hours, a resident came in and probably had no idea what he was getting into taking on a nurse like Justine.

"I want to have a look at his numbers," he said politely as he took the chart.

"I hope you're going to look at the patient, too," Justine shot back.

After reviewing Mr. Housden's chart, the resident stood at the patient's bedside, staring up at the cardiac monitor, thinking out loud. "His pressure is low and his heart is beating fast and irregularly. We need to give him fluids and maybe shock his heart back into a normal sinus rhythm. He may be intravascularly depleted. He looks dry."

"He's not dry, he's dying." Justine held her patient's hand and looked at him in dismay and then glared at the resident with disdain. "This poor man is trying to die."

"Yes, and I'm trying to figure out what's wrong with him."

"I'll tell you what's wrong with him. His diagnosis is imminent death from old age."

"Yes, and there's a chance we can save him from that."

"From what? From dying a day or two later?"

"You never know, he might get out of here. We're here to save lives, aren't we?"

"These heroics are cowardly."

"This man is probably someone's loved one." With his fingers he landmarked the man's neck in the place he planned to insert a central line. Should he try for the subclavian vein and probably win praise from the staff physician or go for the easier internal jugular?

"I hope no one ever loves me this much," Justine said bitterly.

A few hours later, after lots of drugs and electric shocks to his heart, they managed to get the patient's heart in a slower, regular rhythm, but now his blood pressure was low.

"The systolic is still in the double-digits," said Justine, taking it manually with a blood pressure cuff. She went off in search of Old Father Powers who made rounds in the ICU every evening. He had watery blue eyes and big black glasses that always slipped down his nose as he checked the patient board for Catholic-sounding names. He jotted them down and then blessed the whole board of names, just to be on the safe side. Justine went over and gave him a bear hug. "The chaplain was here earlier for another patient and now you, Father," Justine said. "Is the big guy gonna show up next?" The priest chuckled but as he drew closer to the patient, he became solemn. "Is he alive, Justine?"

"He's hanging in there, Father, just barely. He must be waiting for you."

"This is going to give the wrong impression," the resident whispered to Justine while the priest administered last rites.

"Which is what?" Even Justine could be made incredulous.

"If the family shows up, it'll make them think he's not going to make it."

Justine looked at the blood pressure at eighty systolic, his heart rate fast and irregular. She ignored him.

The resident got hold of a nephew over the phone and by default (as there were no other contenders), he became "next of kin." He hadn't been in touch with his uncle for years and said he wouldn't be able to come and see him. "Please do everything you can for him. He's a great guy."

We'd seen every type of family: families who came every day and those who didn't come at all. There were families who didn't wish to be present at the time of death and those who wanted to be there *only* at the time of death. Some families called in frequently, but couldn't bear to visit. Nothing infuriated Justine more than when patients died alone.

But this time Justine was fuming about more than that. "It is inconceivable that someone would die of natural causes!" she exploded at the resident when he came back from speaking to the nephew.

"But we can do something for this guy. We can fix his cardiac rhythm and if he's got pneumonia we can give him antibiotics. We can cure that. He may also have congestive heart failure, so we can give him a diuretic to pull off fluid and decrease his central venous pressure."

"Say, are we doing all of this for you to get in lots of practice so that when someone we can really save comes in, you'll know what you're doing? Is that it?" Justine wanted to know.

"Try thinking outside of the box." The resident started gathering together the supplies he would need to put in a central line, because he could see Justine wasn't going to help him. "Don't write him off because he's old. Doesn't he deserve a chance?"

"Every organ in his body is shutting down, including his brain! DNR* is not some sinister plot to deal with the sick and infirm. Sometimes it's the kindest thing." She stomped off to cool down at the nurses' station, leaving him to do the central line insertion on his own. Later, when it was time to give her patient his antibiotic, Justine headed over instead to the huge box of pastries at the nurses' station left there by a grateful family, syringe in hand. "I'm going to inject it into this blueberry Danish. At least it'll improve its nutritional content because it's certainly not going to do my patient any good," she said. Of course she didn't go ahead with that outrageous plan, but returned to her patient and gave the drug as ordered. At the end of the shift, I found her sitting beside her patient's bed, looking despondent. "I hate seeing people suffer unnecessarily. I hate keeping the dead alive."

We tried to cheer her up. Laura reminded her that at least it was better than the family that requested we keep their elderly grandmother alive until after her grandson's bar mitzvah and only then withdraw treatment, or the woman who wanted us to maintain her husband on life support just so that she could continue to collect his pension cheques.

Mr. Housden lasted two more days until life support was withdrawn and he died alone.

These situations upset us all and we each have to deal with them. That was Justine's turn and I was positive I saw something change in her that day. As it turned out, not long after that she made the decision to leave the ICU and a few years later left nursing altogether.

---

* Do Not Resuscitate.

MRS. ROSE GREEN was an Orthodox Jew, and I was assigned to be her nurse more frequently than any of the others. The nurses in charge must have figured I would have a special connection with her or that I'd understand her better than the others. I did come to understand her but it wasn't easy. I had to work at it.

Mrs. Green was in her mid-sixties and had five children. Her husband and sons wore long black coats and hats and had side curls and long beards. They stood at the foot of her bed, swaying back and forth as they recited psalms of healing and prayers that called upon the "Great Resuscitator" to bring about a "renewal of body, a renewal of spirit." For years, Rose had suffered from lupus, a disease of the auto-immune system, and consequently developed diabetes and chronic obstructive pulmonary disease (COPD). Despite a dysfunction in almost every organ system in her body, she coped as best she could, kept active, and managed to stay out of the hospital until eventually she was admitted to the ICU in respiratory distress and kidney failure. We got her through that crisis but a few months later she returned, this time requiring a longer period of dependency on the ventilator. Her chronic illness continued to flare up for the next two years, with the intervals at home getting shorter and the ICU stays getting longer and more difficult.

"Ha Shem wants me to live," she told me during one of those stays in the ICU. She used the general term "the Name" as she would never use the actual word or write it any way other than in short form, as "G-d," because if that piece of paper were destroyed, it would be a defilement. "It's not up to me," she said with a shrug of her shoulders. "I am here to serve Him."

A year earlier she had been diagnosed with breast cancer. It had spread to her lungs and she underwent a mastectomy and had chemotherapy. "Now, I have two reasons to wear a wig," she confided in me. It was a comment she probably wouldn't have made to other nurses, but she knew I'd understand that the wig or scarf that she always already wore was a sign of her religious observance, a symbol of her modesty. A woman's hair was only to be viewed by her husband. When she was well enough, we talked about many things. Most of our patients are unconscious or just too sick to converse with us to the extent that I could with Mrs. Green, and

I relished the opportunity. I also sensed she liked having me as her nurse because it gave her the opportunity to explain the importance of the woman's role in keeping a kosher home and welcoming the Sabbath on Friday evenings with the lighting and blessing of the candles. She herself could not light real candles while in the hospital because of the fire hazard, but electric candlesticks were plugged in for her at the precise moment of sunset so she could recite the blessing and they were not to be touched until sunset the following evening. When she was well enough, she could eat but was suspicious of the food provided by the hospital. The label that read "Kosher Style" upset her.

"Food is kosher or not." She pushed the tray away. "One can't be a little pregnant, *nu?*"

"What's *unkosher* about clear fluids?" I picked up the can of ginger ale, the bowl of broth.

"Jell-O, for example, is never kosher." She pointed at the offending plastic cup. "Gelatine comes from horses, an unkosher animal because it does not regurgitate its cud and has an uncloven hoof. Even juice may contain particles of unkosher substances or may not have been properly prepared in a kosher facility."

"Why is there such a preoccupation about food?" It was something I'd always wanted to know.

"Keeping kosher elevates the daily act of eating into a spiritual experience."

I thought of how often I grabbed something to eat in the car or stood with the refrigerator door open, in search of a snack. Mrs. Green explained that by keeping kosher one is reminded of the efforts that went into preparing the food and how the kosher method of slaughtering was humane and paid respect to the life of an animal that is providing sustenance to human beings. Through the mundane, we understand the holy, she explained. Through the daily, we connect with the eternal. "When I was a little girl, if I dropped a slice of bread on the floor, my mother taught me to pick it up and say a blessing. Bread is a symbol of life, and we must always show respect for life above all else."

Mrs. Green survived crisis after crisis and numerous resuscitations, but each recovery actually turned out to be a setback because

it left her in a worsened physical condition. Her body was deteriorating, but her mind was fully lucid and intact. In fact, the very
first thing she did upon opening her eyes every morning was to
begin to move her lips in recitation of her daily prayers of gratitude and thanksgiving, to the "True Judge and Redeemer." On
more than one occasion she stated her wishes unequivocally. She
wanted doctors and nurses to do everything possible, each and
every time, to bring her back to life.

"Even if that quality of life is compromised?" a resident asked
her.

"Who is to decide what is an acceptable quality of life?" she
asked in the Talmudic style of answering a question with a question. "How can *any* life be deemed not worth living?"

Here, finally, was someone who could tell us what she wanted.
To me, privately, she added, "He keeps bringing me back, doesn't
he? I was dead and he revived me. Ha Shem took me right to the
edge and said no, go back. There must be a reason."

The only authority she answered to was the word of "Ha
Shem," as interpreted by the scholars who wrote the Talmud. She
and her husband, Mordecai, consulted daily with their personal
Rabbi and relied on him to interpret the laws they lived by.

Mrs. Green continued to have numerous admissions to the ICU
and each time, I was assigned to her care. I didn't mind, but it did
present me with certain challenges the other nurses didn't have to
face. One quiet Saturday morning in particular, I was doubled with
two stable patients, Mrs. Green and the patient in the room beside
hers. I sensed Mrs. Green wanted to ask me for something but was
hesitant. "Everything okay?" I asked her.

"Could you please ask Noreen to make me a cup of tea?"

I reminded her that I was her nurse and would make it for her
myself.

"No. If Noreen is too busy, please ask Tracy to do it for me."

"Just a minute while I finish giving these meds," I said, "and
I'll plug in the kettle." Why was she so impatient? Then I understood. According to her beliefs, I would be desecrating the Sabbath
by boiling water, thereby using energy to transform matter. Even
opening the refrigerator for the milk and inadvertently activating

the light bulb inside was prohibited on the Sabbath. She would be transgressing by causing me to sin on her behalf, I explained to Tracy, who made the tea.

The next morning, I was taken aback when her night nurse told me that the Rabbi had visited her, late at night after sundown, at the end of the Sabbath. "He asked her for a donation to the synagogue. He said he would say extra prayers for her and asked for a cheque for that, too."

"I guess she can spend her money this way," I said slowly, thinking it over.

"Yeah, but I don't feel right about it," the other nurse said, and explained her uneasiness. "She's vulnerable. It's like she's at his mercy. The Rabbi was worried that her cheque might not be accepted at the bank, so he wanted me to witness her signature, but I refused."

"Yes, it does sound like they might be preying on her, as well as praying for her," I agreed. "It doesn't sit right with me, either."

"She's angry at me for not signing and feels her independence has been taken away. She told me you would sign it because you're Jewish, too."

But Mrs. Green didn't get a chance to speak with me about the matter because that day, once again, her condition suddenly worsened. This time her heart went into atrial fibrillation that caused her blood pressure to drop. We had to shock her heart many times that day and eventually managed to bring it back to a normal sinus rhythm. But there were ominous beats on the monitor, and I brought the crash cart into the room, just in case.

During rounds, Dr. Sandor put out a question that made us all think. Which was the bigger fear if we were to be hospitalized – that too much would be done or too little? That we would be over-treated with unnecessary tests and procedures or under-treated and important things missed? Most of the doctors said too little and most of the nurses said too much. Perhaps we trusted the system more than we should, but if so, then they, not enough.

Dr. Sandor has always been committed to making us scrupulously accountable in our practice. He has raised many questions over the years as well as a few eyebrows. He infuriates us, challenges us, and always makes us think. "Do you remember Mrs. Ford?" I asked him recently.

"That was an important case." He looked at me intently to assess if I realized just how important.

It had happened years ago when I was still fairly new to the ICU but even then I recognized its significance. Mrs. Ford was a sixty-five-year-old woman with ALS[*], also called Lou Gehrig's disease, a slow, debilitating neurological disease that left her body paralyzed, but her mind awake. She was "locked-in," unable to move or speak, yet fully aware of her situation. Dr. Sandor told her she could choose the date and time of her death. Her family gathered around her bed. She said goodbye to everyone. We started a morphine infusion until she was drowsy and at the same time slowly decreased the ventilator settings and the oxygen until she became comatose and then died.

"How were we able to do that for her?" I asked. To this day, I've never really understood it. It seemed so radical to assist a patient to choose the day and conditions of her death and to watch her go from fully awake to drowsy, to unresponsive, to dead in a matter of hours.

Dr. Sandor calmly explained. "In the case of Mrs. Ford's death, we were, as always, guided by the patient's wishes. At all times, we kept uppermost in mind the reasons we were giving the narcotic and we stayed focused on our goal of maintaining the patient's dignity and comfort."

"I'M CONCERNED THAT your patient is allowing a religious authority to make decisions for her," Dr. Sandor expressed to me privately, after rounds, away from Mrs. Green's bedside. We were sitting at a long boardroom table in the glassed-in fishbowl, a.k.a. the "think-tank" behind the nurses' station.

"She did express her wishes, when she was last able to communicate," I said.

---

[*] Amyotrophic lateral sclerosis.

"Yes, but are they truly hers or is she abdicating her autonomy to the Rabbi?"

What I had finally figured out was that Mrs. Green did not believe in the hallowed concept of individual autonomy. To her, religious law had the utmost importance, far greater than a human's puny will or personal preference. We had to back right off, but not until Dr. Sandor gave it one more try. He had to ascertain that these were indeed Mrs. Green's wishes. There wasn't much time left. We both knew that the next crisis was imminent.

We went back out to speak with Mr. Green. The Rabbi stood with him outside Mrs. Green's room. They did not wish to meet with the rest of the team in the "quiet room," but would only stand outside Mrs. Green's room and talk with Dr. Sandor, with me listening in. I understood that they would never speak to me directly, as it is forbidden for a man to address a woman other than one's wife. The Rabbi stated his position to Dr. Sandor. "The Jewish view is that we are to be wise and prudent stewards of our bodies," he explained, palms open, his hands outstretched. "It is our greatest endowment from Ha Shem."

"It is not medically indicated to offer anything further to your wife," Dr. Sandor said to Mr. Green, crossing his arms across his chest and widening his stance. "There is no chance for survival should she have another cardiac arrest."

The Rabbi spoke. "If there is a straightforward and obvious treatment, it must be carried out."

"We do not wish to impose harmful, painful procedures upon your wife," Dr. Sandor said, again to Mr. Green, "because, first of all, they won't be of any benefit and second, it would be inhumane to do so."

"Some tortures are worth enduring," the Rabbi said gently.

I watched Dr. Sandor as the Rabbi spoke. He looked good, and fit, but he'd aged. This work had aged us both. He continued, still addressing Mr. Green. "In my medical opinion it would be wrong and useless to attempt to resuscitate your wife if she experiences another cardiac arrest."

"Is she is on life support?" the Rabbi asked.

"Yes. If any of the machines or medications she is on were to be removed, she would die."

"Is she receiving sedation? She needs to be alert enough to hear the prayers."

Dr. Sandor tried to hide his exasperation. "The main point here is that we need to clarify the plan in the event of a cardiac arrest. My opinion is there is no medical reason to perform CPR on your wife. It will not benefit her in any way."

"Are you saying there is no possibility whatsoever that it would bring her back?" the Rabbi asked.

"It is highly unlikely."

"But didn't you say she has pneumonia? Can't that be cured with antibiotics? Hasn't she recovered from similar crises before? Are you basing your recommendations on what *you* would want? It is not within our moral jurisdiction to decide if a life has no quality, or is not worth living." The Rabbi pursed his lips in consternation and glanced at me. "We, the Jewish people, believe in a sacred reverence for all life. Even this nurse knows that."

This was my chance to jump into the fray. I glanced at Mr. Green and he averted his eyes and turned to the Rabbi, who looked at Dr. Sandor. "From what I understand, *Halacha* – Jewish law – prohibits us from shortening the life, but what does it say about prolonging it unnecessarily?"

"You should know better, Tilda," he said, and invoked again the highest imperative, which is the rescue of a human life, something to be attempted at all costs.

Finally, I was beginning to get it. To them, suffering was worth it for even another moment of life. Mr. Green's wishes, his wife's wishes, were irrelevant. All that mattered were the wishes of "Ha Shem" as the Rabbi understood them.

"Regardless of what we do or don't do, Mrs. Green is going to die," Dr. Sandor said.

"That is not for you to decree." The Rabbi turned and walked away and Mr. Green followed after him. I stood alone in the hall with Dr. Sandor. It is sometimes hard to read his feelings, but there was no mistaking them now; after that encounter, he looked sad.

"Aha," I said, putting my arm around him, "you *do* have feelings. I just saw them." I detected a tiny smile. "You know what, Imré, I have come around to your point of view. I think there are times when what we do is futile."

"I'm shocked, Tilda! I thought you didn't believe in the f-word," he teased me back.

"Perhaps the antidote to futility is meaning. If something has meaning to someone, that redeems it."

"Well, you're too late in coming around, Tilda. Ethicists don't even use the term *futile* any more because it is too value-laden and open to interpretation. We differentiate between physiological futility and quality of life futility," he explained, always the teacher.

"I understand the Green family now," I said, eager to draw to an end this complicated discussion, "but it's still hard to be her nurse."

It was during that fifth ICU admission that Mrs. Green had a final cardiac arrest. We were unable to revive her after a resuscitation attempt that went on for more than two hours, during which we did everything we could until there was nothing left to do. But at least, all the time that we were trying, we felt resolved about what we were doing as we knew that these were her wishes.

"We must not tamper with the soul," she told me in one of her last moments. "Quality of life is not the issue. Life is the most important thing."

MY UNDERSTANDING of Mrs. Green's choice helped me accept it. I also had a deeper understanding of Mrs. Ford's. However, just when I thought I was getting a handle on these complex moral, ethical, and spiritual matters, I heard a story that raised new questions. I was walking past the nurses' station when Louise saw me and called out, "Hey, Tilda!" Louise must be fifty, but yoga classes and good genes make her look thirty. Petite and delicate, she leaned over the countertop and grabbed my hands with surprising strength. "Have I got a story for you!" Who had time for stories? It was insanely busy and who should know that better than Louise herself who was in charge of the ICU that day? We

were short six nurses, and patients were being admitted and transferred out all day. I assumed she would tell me the story later, if
we managed to get a coffee break.

"I've got to tell you now," she insisted, pencilling a name in the
staffing book and then setting it aside.

I motioned to someone to cover for me, that I'd be back to
my room in a minute or two, and leaned over the counter
with my elbows resting on the ledge. Louise's eyes locked with
mine and held fast.

"You'll want to get this down," she said, her eyes sparkling. She
could hardly contain herself.

I reached over the countertop to grab a few scraps of paper that
our ward clerk leaves for us to record lab results and telephone
numbers. "Shoot," I said, my pen poised. As she began to speak,
it grew quiet around us. Tracy took over Louise's work for her.
Other nurses moved closer to listen and others moved out of the
way as if to clear a path for this story to be told.

"Has it ever happened to you, Tilda, that you love a friend's
mother like your own?"

"Yes." I thought about Bunny, Joy's mother, and other bor-
rowed mothers, both past and present. I felt a swell of all the
mother love they had offered me and all that I felt for them.

"You remember I told you about Alice? She's my best friend
Meredith's mother. I loved her like my own mother. Last year she
was diagnosed with lung cancer and I made a promise to her that
I would help her when the time came." I nodded. "Oh, I wish you
had known her! She was brilliant and very strong-minded. She
read everything – you'd have loved her, Tilda. But during her last
year, she struggled to breathe and couldn't get around. She had no
appetite and lost forty pounds. One day she told me all she wanted
was a cigarette, just one. She already had lung cancer, so why
couldn't she have one? She enjoyed it so much. She had a right to
that bit of enjoyment, don't you think?" We nodded and Louise
took a deep breath and closed her eyes to help her find her place
in the story again. "A few days ago, Meredith called me. Her
mother was in distress and they took her to the hospital. Alice said,

'It's time. I want Louise here. She'll know what to do.' I said to Meredith on the phone, 'Just don't let them start feeding her. And no intubation.' Then I got in my car and booted it up there. I was going so fast, the police stopped me but when I explained why they let me go. Alice was so relieved to see me. 'Can we do this?' she asked, and I told her, yes. Of course by that time she had a feeding tube in place and the crash cart right by her bed. Oh, it drives me crazy, Tilda! Not every person needs CPR before they die!"

I nodded and reached over for a few more of those little slips of paper to get all of this down.

"Well, Alice was very anxious and having difficulty breathing. She was on a self-controlled pain medication pump, but I think she was too stressed to use it, so the first thing I did was push the pump for her and then I asked to have the dose increased. Soon, she drifted off to sleep. A doctor came in and asked why she was so out of it. He said they were taking her for a CT scan and then a pleural tap to drain the fluid in her lungs, but Alice had already told them she didn't want any more procedures or interventions. 'Who's the one with some medical background?' the doctor growled. He must have sensed a threat. I waved my hand to show I was the guilty party. 'I'm an ICU nurse, for twenty years.' He asked if Alice was still smoking. Alice heard that and pulled off her oxygen mask to ask me, 'Do you think it would have made a difference if I had stopped smoking?' I told her, 'Why take this with you? You loved smoking. You had a wonderful life. Let it go.'" Louise rolled her eyes. "I arranged to have Alice transferred to a palliative care unit. Oh, it was beautiful there and we could all be with her. Alice asked me to make it happen faster. I would never do that, but I had to find the balance between keeping her comfortable and not speeding up her dying."

"Louise, phone's for you," the ward clerk interrupted. "It's the OR. The patient is coming out in twenty minutes. Will the bed be ready?"

She nodded. We all knew she'd be returning to her efficient, responsible self in a couple of moments, but there were still a few details she had to tell. "Alice looked at me and gave me that stare. You've seen it, right?"

"You mean the one right before?" I asked, and Louise nodded.

"She looked right at me and asked, 'How will I know when I'm dead?' Tilda, it was extraordinary. It had been an overcast day, but at that moment, the sun broke out of the clouds and Alice's bed was filled with sunlight. She looked like an angel lying there and I knew exactly what to say: 'Alice, you'll know you're dead when you're looking down at us.'"

We were in a frieze of reposes, still and quiet, listening with our entire bodies.

"Alice looked me in the eye and said, 'I'm dying, aren't I?' I said, 'Yes, Alice, you are.' It was the most amazing thing to see someone completely aware, experiencing her own death. She was saying goodbye and beginning the journey of leaving us behind. She was excited. She believed she was going on to something else and she was not afraid. I had promised her I'd keep her pain-free and comfortable and I did that. She was aware right up until the moment when she wasn't aware any more. I thank my lucky stars I had the skills to be able to help her.

"Then she started Cheyne-Stoking, with gasps and long pauses and then another gasp and a pause. The family was distressed at her breathing, but I explained that this was natural and expected."

I've seen how the "death rattle" unnerves many people, even some nurses. It is raw, animal-like, and different from any other sound on earth. Many interpret it as a cry of distress, but when experienced nurses hear it, they feel a sense of peace and relief. They know the person is unconscious, feels no pain, and that the end is near. The families are grieving, so nurses turn their attention to them. I've seen families become desperate to have a fast transition from life to death, like what they've seen on hospital TV shows. They can't handle the lingering passage in between. They want it over with quickly.

"The pauses got longer and then stopped. I put my ear to her chest and told them she was gone."

"Wow," everyone murmured. We'd seen many deaths but never one like that. In the ICU we are so reliant on machines to tell us when the moment has arrived. Most of us had not seen a death unmediated by technology.

Louise smiled. "At the funeral, the minister came over to me. 'Ah, so you were the nurse who helped Alice in her last hours,' he said. It was the proudest moment of my life."

I DON'T THINK you could work in the ICU for any length of time and not think about your own death. Recently, I told Dr. Sandor my wishes in the event that I become critically ill.

"What about organ donation?" he asked.

"Yes, I want to donate my organs."

"Tissues, too?"

Consistency and clarity decrease confusion, he's always said. I hesitated momentarily, fleetingly recalling what Casey once told me. She said she would donate everything except her corneas. "I know it sounds weird," she chuckled, "but I don't want to be blind on the journey, wherever it is that I am going."

But I felt differently. "Yes, all of my organs and tissues, too."

"What about burial of the remains?"

"No, no burial." *He doesn't mess around!*

"Cremation, then?"

No, I told him about biodegradable internments I'd been reading about, about the body disintegrating, becoming fertilizer and rejoining the ecosystem.

"But isn't that against your religion?"

Good question. I am still trying to figure out what I believe, but I am Jewish and Jews have been doing eco-friendly burials for years. Yom Kippur, the holiest day in the Jewish calendar, is supposed to be a *death rehearsal* when Jews fast and wear white just like the plain cotton shrouds that they are to be buried in. But even if one doesn't have a religion, doesn't everyone have something they believe in? Last spring, when it seemed like just about everyone was celebrating something, a feast, a festival, or a fast of Ramadan, Easter, Passover, or Diwali, I asked Boris, a hospital assistant who immigrated to Canada from secular, Communist Russia what he celebrated.

"Nothing," he answered in his serious, but sweet way.

"Do you celebrate May Day, International Workers' Day?" I tried.

"No, not any more."

"What, then?"

"March 8 is the only day I celebrate," he said with an impish grin.

"What's that?"

"International Women's Day."

How could I forget?

But it finally all made sense to me last December 25 when I arrived for a day shift just as Ibrahim, another of our hospital assistants, was heading home after his night shift.

"Merry Christmas," he called out to me with a wave.

"Merry Christmas to you, too."

After all, isn't the *true* spirit of Christmas what we all share? Perhaps it will be through the universal bond of values – justice, forgiveness, goodwill, and compassion – which all the great religions have in common, that Muslims like him and Jews like me can find the way to greet each other in peace.

10

COMFORT MEASURES

It is only with the heart that one can see rightly; what is essential is invisible to the eye.

— Antoine de Saint-Exupéry

Today, twenty years after starting in the ICU, I call it home. To me, the work is just as challenging, exciting, fascinating, and at times, fun. But there are still situations that continue to puzzle and perplex me. Take what happened just the other week.

After nearly three hours of non-stop activity, I finally emerged from my patient's room. Mr. Rodriguez was a middle-aged father of two who had had a liver transplant two days prior. After a rocky forty-eight hours, there were now hopeful signs that his new liver was working. However, he was still on maximum ventilator support and unconscious. I had given him a bath, a shave, shampoo, back rub, and changed his bed linen. I made adjustments to his medications, gave him an antibiotic, observed his respirations, checked the ventilator, measured his central venous pressure, pulmonary artery pressures, and cardiac output, and compared all of these numbers against previous readings, and made additional adjustments to his medications. I went into the tiny anteroom outside the patient's and stripped off my gown, gloves, mask, and goggles that we all had to wear to curtail dissemination of the bacterial infection he'd acquired while in hospital. I washed my hands, sat down at my computer to begin my charting, all the while keeping my eyes on my patient and the cardiac monitor. I was just about to take a sip of the coffee I'd bought earlier when several visitors happened to walk past and I overheard one say to the other, "See how the nurses sit outside the room? That way they don't have to go to the patients as much."

"Yeah, *right*. All we do is sit here," I grumbled under my breath, but apparently not softly enough, because she heard me and turned back.

"Oh, I'm sorry, dear. I'm sure you are all working very hard."

"No, *I'm* sorry," I said, and we both fell over each other apologizing again, she for her offhand comment and me for my sarcastic retort. But it's easy to see how she could get the impression we were doing nothing. Much of nursing care is invisible, especially to the casual observer. So many things we do are private and extremely intimate and take place behind closed doors or drawn curtains. And those "comfort measures," the repositioning, those gentle, reassuring touches, the hugs, the understanding of things unsaid, the back rubs – and more – seem simple and trivial, especially when compared to the big-ticket items doctors offer, such as tests and prescriptions.

"Why do you bathe patients so much?" a student nurse once asked me. "It's not like they're dirty."

"It feels good to patients," I explained to her. "Water is relaxing and it makes a person feel fresh and clean." The hospital had been trying to get us to use new antibacterial "bath in a bag" chemical wipes, but nothing was better than water. In fact, I had been working on an invention for a portable shower contraption that could be placed over the bed and would rain down warm water all over the patient. The water will drip off all the sides, into troughs, but I hadn't got around to building the prototype just yet.

Researchers measure, quantify, document, describe, evaluate, in order to validate nursing and prove its effectiveness, but something seems to get lost in the process. Data is generated and numbers are crunched but the essence, beyond the tasks and skills, continues to elude scientists. Cardiac monitoring is one of those particularly invisible activities. It looks like nothing more than blank staring, or casual gazing, but it is actually a studied vigilance that requires a deep understanding of the heart's electrical system, the skill to identify a potentially lethal problem, and the knowledge to intervene. While the attention required looks incidental and easy, the thinking behind it is anything but: *why has the heart rate jumped from 80 to 110? Is he in pain? Is he "dry" and needs a fluid bolus? I better take his temperature . . . fever can cause the heart to race. What's his hemoglobin? What about those premature atrial contractions? Are they causing a compromise in blood pressure? And those ventricular contractions, are they unifocal or multifocal? I'll check his potassium level because if it's low, that's what could be causing an arrhythmia.*

Those aspects of nursing that are elusive, indefinable, and ambiguous contribute to a debate that rages not only within the insular walls of the institutes of education, but also in the real-life places where nursing is practised: What is a nurse? That is, what are the roles, responsibilities, and actions that define a nurse? Who is a nurse? That is, what does a nurse look like and how can you tell one apart from the doctor or other professionals? More worrisome is that patients have been known to ask, "How can I tell who is my nurse?" given that gender and clothing alone are not definitive. Most nurses say they wish to be known by the relationships they have with patients, not by their clothes. I've seen many nurses individualize their uniforms by wearing scrubs in ice-cream colours of raspberry, lemon, and grape. There are those who wear lab coats decorated with teddy bears, angels, or lollipops.

Later that day after the incident with the visitor passing by, I decided to ask some of the other nurses sitting in the lounge about clothes. "Do you remember Carrie? The one who tied her scrubs with a gold lamé belt and always wore a string of pearls? What a *fashionista* she was!"

"I remember her," someone recalled with a chuckle. "That girl really knew how to pimp her uniform. She wore those white shoes with the kitten heels that went clickety-clack down the hall. You could always hear her coming. And what about her nail art? She had those long, curved acrylic ones and when she was dating that sailor she decorated them with nautical symbols! I always meant to ask how she managed to insert a catheter. *Ouch*!"[*]

"Why do we even have to wear uniforms?" someone else asked. "We're individuals, aren't we?"

"In the old days," reminisced Phyllis, a senior nurse, still going strong in our physically taxing work, "we worked hard for our caps and white uniforms and when you put them on, you felt like a real nurse. It was like you were preparing for your role in a play. It meant something."

Monica kept quiet, but I felt certain she had a strong opinion on the matter. I knew her ambitions. Even with a young daughter who she supports on her own and after going through a messy divorce, Monica has returned to school for her Master's degree in management and is a stellar student. Finally, she spoke up. "Appearance matters. How would you feel if the pilot of the plane you're on showed up wearing track pants and a T-shirt? What kind of impression would that make? And what about all the bling nurses are wearing these days? It doesn't look professional and surely they know jewellery harbours bacteria that we can bring in or take home with us." A chorus of dissent flared up, but Monica continued above the din. "Besides, the hospital has a dress code and we're supposed to adhere to it."

"That's just a way for management to control us. It takes away our individuality!"

"What's a nurse supposed to look like?"

Someone sarcastically offered the suggestion, "Try the 'Naughty Nurse' website. You can get some wild ideas there!"

"My kids want to dress up as nurses for Halloween. What can they wear to look like a nurse?"

"Have you seen that nurse in Dialysis who still wears a cap? What a dinosaur!"

---

[*] I didn't get a chance to tell them about Justine's famous T-shirts, like the one that reads: "Nurses Call the Shots" imprinted over a scary-looking needle and syringe. Then there was a night she wore one that said, "Institute for the Sexually Gifted" and handed out fake "Virgin Restorer Pills" to the older nurses, who laughed about it until the morning.

"Did you see that doctor who came to see my patient this morning? He looked like a geeky high school student, no lab coat, no name tag, nothing. He went into my patient's chart. Who are you, I asked him? He looked like he'd walked in off the street. He could have been a visitor or a patient from the Psych ward!"

Nurses' uniforms seem to be yet another issue in the ongoing debate about what and who a nurse is. Uniforms did have a way of obliterating individuality. They could turn people into a service to such a degree that ease of recognition or the speed with which they responded to a call bell became the measure of their worth. Even I, who always preferred the generic, unisex, and equalizing qualities of my green or blue scrubs, recently purchased a pair of shiny, candy-apple red shoes for work, as much for the vibrant colour as for the comfort. Is individual expression really such a threat? Can't beauty and function coexist? What if nurses could find ways to use Beauty and Art as capably as they use Science?

I was pondering all of this one day at the grocery store. While I realize most people start at the produce sections, move on to refrigerated items and frozen foods last, I head straight to the jumbled bin of remaindered or damaged books. I was digging in there and happened to dredge out a book of unexpected possibility: *Transitions: Unlocking the Creative Quilter Within*, by Andrea Balosky, a Californian quilter. I stood there, entranced. Wow, I thought, looking at photographs of her quilts. The juxtapositions of shapes and colours thrilled me! The mix of vintage and modern! The artistic and the functional! That book sparked my exploration of quilt history and lore. Even the names of traditional blocks intrigued me: Flying Geese, Log Cabin, Broken Dishes, Hidden Windows, Jacob's Ladder, Card Trick, and Courthouse Steps. I loved the "crazy quilts" that didn't use uniform shapes and instead had a distinctive haphazard look. There were equally lovable scrap quilts with mismatched, chaotic colours and glaring, but appealing, flaws. Other quilts, such as in the Amish style, were balanced, symmetrical, and in muted colours. Many quilters used whatever was on hand; their intention was not perfection. Quilts have even found a place in museums as examples of both simple folk art and sophisticated craftwork.

An idea was brewing . . .

Inspiration can come from unexpected places. A fortune cookie once did it for me. "You have the power to affect the quality of someone's day." Nurses have that power in ways that are both obvious and practical but also subtle, even spiritual. And it's not only nurses who have that opportunity, I discovered one morning when I rode the elevator with the housekeeping staff, who start their day as early as nurses. A cadre of Portuguese and Italian ladies in pink smocks got on at the basement floor, each one carrying a plastic bag containing a mop head. "They give us a clean one to start each day," one lady told me with obvious pride. "We used to have to wash them ourselves at home, but now the hospital does it for us. Some of the girls weren't cleaning them properly," she said, showing her disapproval of such sloppy practice. "It's so nice to start the day with a fresh mop."

And none of us will forget the sweet voice of the young man who worked the evening switchboard. We stopped whatever we were doing at precisely 2100 hours to listen to the public announcement:

> Good evening, ladies and gentlemen. This is a gentle reminder that it is now nine o'clock and the time has come to say goodnight to those you love. It's a cold one out there this evening, around five degrees, but it's more like minus twenty with the windchill factor. Brrr . . . We suggest you bundle up with a hat and scarf to keep warm. Have a safe journey home. We'll be looking forward to seeing you again tomorrow when you are welcome to visit us again. Goodbye and sweet dreams. Be well. Take care of yourselves and we'll take good care of the patients.

We looked at each other, amazed. How long could he get away with it? As it turned out, not long. The public announcement soon reverted to the original, terse recorded message: "Visiting hours are now over."

I WAS BEGINNING to piece together a patchwork of ideas. What if a collective of nurses created a work of art made out of natural elements such as cotton, wool, and paint in this environment of chrome, glass, steel, plastic, and concrete? A nurses' patchwork quilt, made by our hands, those very hands that do the work of caring for our patients? It would be inspired both by what is in our hearts and our minds. It could be a symbol of comfort, a soft place to rest one's eyes, especially the anxious, weary ones of our visitors out in the waiting room where it could eventually be hung and displayed.

I called a meeting of all the nurses. I took a deep breath as I opened a big plastic storage box and pulled out pens, paints, crayons, tubes of glitter, ribbon, and squares of plain white fabric. They looked at me, some dubious, others bemused, and a few annoyed. I explained my idea.

"There she goes again," they groaned, rolling their eyes, "another of her crazy make-work projects."

"Who does she think we are? A bunch of grannies?"

"Yeah, *my* grandmother makes quilts, too."

"The time has come to appreciate these historic domestic arts, not trivialize them," I lectured. "You're buying into the usual putdown of women's work." (Funny, how it wasn't any of the male nurses who objected to the quilt.) "It's because we have come so far that we can feel proud of art created by our hands. It doesn't stereotype us any more."

They weren't convinced. Many walked out, laughing as they went. To the remaining ones, I turned up the heat a notch. "It will be a place to put our stories, our memories and save them from extinction. Nursing might look different in the years to come. This quilt will be a statement of our profession, a historical document of nursing today, now, in this place and time."

"What's the theme?" someone asked.

"Comfort measures," I came up with on the spot.

"Tilda, do you really think that a quilt can change the world?" someone else asked.

I did, in fact, believe that *Art* could, but kept quiet. They'd heard enough from me. Reluctantly, they took their package of fabric and supplies. A few showed mild interest. But was it such a stretch? Many nurses had creative hobbies of some sort or another. Take Valerie. She's such an accomplished gardener that tour buses stop at her house to visit her garden. She tends to her patients in the same way. She took care of a prisoner who was brought to the hospital from jail where he had taken a heroin overdose. He was ugly and tough and had a tattoo of barbed wire encircling his neck, arms, and chest. A policeman kept a constant watch over him, even though a critically ill patient could hardly escape. I came over to help Valerie because I knew he could be violent. However, in her hands, he was docile.

"What's he in jail for?" I asked the policeman, who was sitting in the room.

"Rape, murder. The usual." He flapped open his newspaper.

The patient/prisoner could not have known, but must have felt, the benefit of Valerie's profound philosophy of nursing that she once expressed to me: "I don't care who you are. I'm going to give you the best care I possibly can. It doesn't take much. It's really so simple. A smile, a kind word. It means so much." Valerie puts her gardening skills to use in other ways, as well. Her patients are always well-tended and their rooms are always clean, orderly, and nice-smelling, if possible. And I am positive that it was Valerie who potted a plant in a bedpan and placed it on the counter of the nursing station for all to enjoy.

There are other professionals who have also found ways to allow their hobbies to inform their work in the ICU. On her days off, Monique, our Québécoise physiotherapist, is an extreme athlete who participates in "adventure" races. She's part of a team that goes four days straight without a break, bushwhacking through wilderness, running through hills and valleys, traversing rivers and streams.

"*Incroyable!*" I said. "What about sleep?"

"I got about three and a half hours on the last one. We took a few naps," she admitted. "It was wild."

"What about food?"

"Energy bars, pre-cooked bacon for the fat. Lots of water, but we have to carry it with us."

Her work with our patients involves assisting them to bend a knee or cough out tenacious secretions lodged in their lungs. She helps them dangle their legs over the side of the bed after a prolonged illness or do breathing exercises after surgery. These are their "Iron Man" events and Monique knows that well. *Bien sur.*

"DOESN'T ANYONE GET BETTER?" friends often ask me. Understandably, they want to hear heartwarming stories. They are tired of my sighs and lamentations about my work. Why have I never told them about Dr. Margaret Herridge's world-renowned work on the long-term survival of patients with ARDS?[*] We took care of those patients only during their stay in the ICU when they were critically ill, but Dr. Herridge follows the growing number of survivors who made it home. She documented their progress as they returned to good health.

Why had I never told anyone about the son, his mother, and the liver they now share? She had a rare disease and only a transplant would save her life. The son worked with his parents in a thriving family business and they had gone on yearly family trips to their native Italy and come back tanned and fit – except for one summer when the mother returned weak and jaundiced. Her subsequent deterioration was rapid. It didn't take long for the son to decide to donate a lobe of his liver to his mother and luckily he was a match. "Imagine this miracle," the mother said, "a son gives birth to his mother!" A nurse brought the son over in a wheelchair from his hospital room on a surgical floor. She helped reach his arms to his mother in the bed while I lifted the mother's arms toward the son. Together we made it possible for the two of them to hug each other.

Why had I never shown my friends or family the calendar put out by the organ donor association? It included pictures of a kidney recipient kayaking in a lake, a liver transplant running a marathon, another smiling, sitting in her garden.

---

[*] Acute Respiratory Distress Syndrome, a life-threatening lung injury that requires a long and difficult course of treatment.

What about that eighteen-year-old boy with testicular cancer that had spread throughout his body, who had a tumour, the size of a football, wrapped around his heart? He underwent surgery but then developed pneumonia and kidney failure and landed up in the ICU. "We couldn't remove all of the tumour," the surgeon told the patient's mother and brother. "We'll have to go back in again once these complications resolve."

"But he's okay?" they asked in unison, rushing ahead of him into the room.

"For now," he said.

"Hey, bud, the doctor said you are okay!" The brother grabbed his brother's hand. "I just about went *boom*, passed out, and Mom's here, freaking right out." Amidst the IV and the arterial line, he found a place to plant a kiss on the back of his brother's hand. "I'd do anything for you, man. You're my main bro. Maybe I'll bring the catcher's mitt, and we can play ball in here."

After the family left the room, I spoke with the surgeon. "He's the sickest patient in the ICU right now," I told him, trying to hide my worry.

"He's young and his type of cancer has an excellent response rate to the chemo plus surgery regimen. We're aiming for total cure. There's no other option." He closed the chart.

"Yes, but he's developed so many problems and he's on maximum support." I gestured around at the room full of machines, including the High-Frequency Jet Ventilator that was used only in extreme cases such as this. It pumps more than 100 breaths into the lungs every minute and makes a loud, rapid, thumping noise you can hear throughout the halls of the ICU.

"He'll be all right. He'll get out of here." The surgeon got up to go. "If you nurses would be more optimistic," he said with exasperation, "the patients would do better."

Maybe it was just a bad day or I had seen too many losses and attended too many "M and M" rounds of late, where the mortality and the morbidity of our patients were reviewed and we spent hours discussing all that had gone wrong and the ways we could do better next time.

"How is he?" said the mother, rushing in later that day in her coat and scarf.

"About the same," I said evenly. "He's holding his own. No better and no worse, but that's saying a lot." *Around this place, it is.*

"Amen," she said, clutching my arm. "Amen."

But the next day, I was able to tell her, "He's getting better," and he was, a little.

"Praise the Lord for this miracle." She clasped her hands up to God in gratitude and then out toward me. "Thank you, Nurse, for everything you are doing for my boy."

We saw that young man again just a few weeks later. Tall and shy-looking, with the requisite baseball cap turned around and baggy pants, he came to visit us under duress from his mother. Was it a miracle or merely an accurate reflection of statistics and the laws of large numbers that bore out the doctor's confident prediction? Sometimes everything went well, not only as prayed and hoped for, but as planned and intended for also. This is what the ICU is about and one of the reasons I work here, yet these are not the stories I regale my friends and family with, when I tell them anything at all. Why don't these stories leave as strong an imprint on my memory or as lasting a residue on my emotions as the ones that disturb me, even *haunt* me at times? I suppose it's because, generally speaking, our patients are the ones with complications; they come to us when things don't go as planned and hoped. The cures and successes aren't the ones who need us or who keep us busy or up late at night.

A NURSE CALLED from the floor one day and I happened to answer the phone. "There's a patient here named Mr. Robichaud who wants you to pay him a visit," she said. "He's doing great after his liver transplant, but he says he has some concerns."

"Me? I didn't take care of a Mr. Robichaud."

"He says any nurse will do. He has questions about his stay in the ICU."

I volunteered to go and another nurse took over my patient while I went to the seventh floor.

"I hear they drugged me," said a wan, worried-looking man in his forties, after I introduced myself. "I lost eight whole days of my life."

"Yes, it must feel like that," I said. "Pain medication was given to you after the surgery. Some of those drugs make you lose your memory for those events, others can distort your thinking."

"Yeah, I can't remember what happened there. I was terrified. All I could think of was if this is my life now, I want to end it. The clock moved so slowly. I couldn't talk and always felt like I was choking because of the tube in my mouth. I panicked when I couldn't see the nurse. Most were nice, but there were a few who were rough."

"I am sorry to hear that," I said quietly.

"But why did they dope me up so much?"

"You were probably in discomfort or pain," I explained, but then tried a different tack. "What do you feel you missed?"

He thought for a moment. "My wife bought the kids a puppy and there was a hurricane in New Orleans . . ." He was incredulous that the world had gone on in his absence. "Wait, there's more . . ."

"Yes? Tell me."

"The morning of my transplant, before I even knew there was a liver for me, I sensed something. The nurses moved differently. They kept stepping out of my room to whisper to each other. The day before, I had been given a meal tray, but that morning, nothing, with no explanation. Hardly anyone spoke to me and when they did it was with these bright, overly cheerful expressions pasted on their faces as if they had a secret." He gave a weak chuckle. "Oh, they had a secret all right. But I didn't dare ask what it was. I had been carrying a pager for two years. One time it went off, but it was a wrong number and that sent me into a tailspin. I'm ashamed to admit how long I'd been praying for some young, healthy person to die. If it was going to happen anyway, why not for me? I was hoping for a car crash, headlong collision preferably, so that the vital internal organs would still be intact." He paused and I sat there until he was ready to say more. "I've always been a light drinker, on social occasions only, or a glass of wine at dinner – doesn't everyone? Haven't done drugs for years, but how I got hepatitis – I have no idea. They say it's idiopathic – no known cause."

"It seems like you are remembering a lot more."

"But not my eight days in the ICU. I've lost all of that." We sat there together for a long while until he spoke again. "I am very grateful for this new chance at life, but it still bothers me what I missed. I'd like to know what happened in the ICU. I have nightmares about it."

"Would it help to visit the ICU?" He nodded eagerly and reached for his dressing gown. Since he was still too weak to walk, I found a wheelchair. As soon as I pressed the metal button to mechanically open the doors of the ICU, he recoiled and covered his eyes with his hands. What was it, I asked, the mere glimpse of the place? The noise? The smells? "Yes, all of those things," he said. "I remember now – too much. Please take me back to my room."

WE SO SELDOM SEE the results of our efforts and no matter what we do to ameliorate the experience, no matter how hard we try to bring about some measure of comfort, the bottom line is that no one wants to be here. It's perfectly understandable that most patients wouldn't want to return to the scene of their pain and suffering. However, it is very sweet when patients do come to visit us, often looking so well that we hardly recognize them. I think of them like soldiers returning from the war, a little stunned and still shaken, but grateful to have survived a mighty battle. We gather around them, keeping a respectful distance and listening to their testimonies.

SOME PATIENTS got better so fast! I had a patient who had a lung transplant and the next morning we extubated her and by that afternoon, she was sitting up in a chair taking sips of water. "You're making amazing progress," I told her.

"It's because I prayed so hard," she explained. "That's the reason I got the lungs so fast. I was only on the list for five days." She put her feet up on the little stool I brought for her and rearranged the blanket over her knees.

"Mmm," I said, trying hard to keep my mind open to what she was saying.

"My doctor said it was a perfect match and everything went smoothly in the operating room. It's because we prayed so much. The whole church prayed for me."

"But what about patients who also pray, just as you did, but things don't go as well for them?"

"They must have lost their faith. They've slipped and wavered or maybe didn't pray hard enough. That's not to say my husband and I are perfect," she admitted. "We're sinners, too."

WE WERE ALMOST at the end of a shift when we got a call from the critical care dispatch centre saying that they were sending us a patient. We raced to prepare the room for someone about whom we knew very little. The mother arrived first, always a bad sign: the patient was likely someone young. She was a nineteen-year-old girl in shock, unconscious, and in fulminant liver failure. We moved her onto the bed, hooked her up to the monitors and the ventilator. Her blood pressure was dangerously low and her lungs were filled with fluid. She was in a coma and bleeding everywhere as her liver had completely stopped working and was unable to produce essential clotting factors. Her mother stood there, gripping a jug of her daughter's urine. She told us her daughter had been out at an all-night rave, had come home that morning and seemed fine. She went to sleep, but didn't get up for her job at the music store in the afternoon, and her mother couldn't wake her. The doctor took her aside and explained that her daughter's liver had inexplicably shut down and that if we could manage to stabilize her condition, we might be able to put her on the transplant list and wait for an organ. He could not tell at this time what caused the liver failure. As the doctor spoke, the mother kept her eyes on us, watching us work on her daughter. I saw her hand move to the place on her own body, feel for it and press in. I read her thoughts: she was ready, at that very moment, to offer up her own liver, if she could.

I finished that shift and then was off work for the next few days. I made a point of not calling in to find out how she was doing, as I

sometimes did. It's enough, I told myself. I have to make that separation. There's a limit to how much I can care – isn't there? But
on the next shift, I came in early. If she was still alive, I wanted to
be her nurse. I looked to her room. There was a Korean man in
her place. *Had they moved her to another room?* I flipped through
the patient logbook. Ms. Celeste Alaya – Transferred to General
Medicine. *The floor? Impossible!* How could she have progressed
from being critically ill to going home in just three days? Perhaps
she had been sent to the floor to die? Sometimes the floor nurses
were more able to provide palliative care in a private room
than we were in the ICU. I saw the resident who had been on that
evening. "What happened to that young girl in liver failure?"
I pointed at the room where she had been.

He thought for a moment. "Oh, her? She got better. We transferred her out." His gaze returned to his computer and he scrolled
down to something on the screen.

"What was it? An overdose? Did she ingest something weird?
Was it hepatitis or an infection from her body piercings? Was it a
tropical disease from her trip to Jamaica?"

"No . . . we never actually arrived at a definitive diagnosis."

"What made her better? Dialysis? Plasmapheresis? Antibiotics?"

"Nothing in particular. None of that." He shrugged a shoulder.
"I guess it was Tincture of Time. You know, old Mother Nature."
He looked off into space. "And nursing care."

Everyone needed a diagnosis, didn't they?

I had to see for myself. I raced up to the floor. The curtain
was closed around the bed and her mother was packing a suit-
case. A pretty young woman pulled open the curtain. "Who's
there, Ma?" She was zipping up her jeans and jiving to a beat on
her iPod.

So, here was another mystery. Just as people could get inexplicably sick, they could also get inexplicably well. But did there have
to be a miraculous recovery in order to have the heart uplifted and
warmed? Some of the most tragic losses I have witnessed were
inspiring for reasons other than recoveries. It's easy to get excited
about success.

A fit young woman, a mother of two, was running a marathon

when she dropped to her knees. She was brought to us, deeply unresponsive, her pupils barely reactive to light. We put her on a heart-lung machine* to oxygenate her blood outside of her body because her lungs couldn't fulfill that function and her heart was so damaged it could not pump adequately. Her blood pressure plummeted despite the maximum dosages of the drugs we gave her. Then, two days later, when she was off ECMO, we took her for an MRI† scan and saw that her brain had become so swollen it bulged down into her spinal cord. She was irretrievable and the doctors deemed further medical treatment to be futile.

As all that was happening, her mother, who lived in England, was flying on a plane to be with her daughter. She arrived during the night and I brought her directly into the ICU, straight to her daughter's bed. The mother took her hand and stood for a long time, taking in the sight of the swollen, motionless body attached to machines whose dancing lines and beeping alarms made it seem more alive than the patient. "Oh, Cat," she moaned, as if her daughter were a little girl, merely misbehaving. Then she turned to me and said, "My Catherine is dead. I see that." She did not want to speak to a doctor or be shown the results of the MRI to prove what she knew as a mother. "I thought it through all the way on the plane," she said softly, "and I accept it. My Cat is gone." We stood together and I felt the vast understanding between us that, although miraculous recoveries were possible, there was no miracle to be had here. I pulled up two chairs and we sat together. After a long while, she spoke. "I want everything turned off." She waved away the machines around her daughter. "I want Cat released from all of this."

"It's only been forty-eight hours," I said. "The doctor wants to speak with you in the morning."

"We're doing this for the doctors?" She smiled as if she pitied them for their inadequate understanding of a mother. "Has a person in this condition ever recovered?"

---

* It is called ECMO for extra-corporeal membrane oxygenation.
† Magnetic resonance imaging is another type of scan, particularly useful for visualizing the brain.

I didn't answer her because I felt she had arrived at her own conclusions, but the thought of having to wait for what she saw as a formality disturbed this otherwise imperturbable mother. "What is the effect on her spirit to be kept in this state of suspension, this limbo between life and death, sustained on chemicals and machines?" Her voice choked and she paused to collect and contain herself. "Anyone can see she's dead. I could hold on to her with my love. You could keep her here with your machines, but it's beyond all of us now. It's out of our hands and I accept it." She, who had much more at stake, was more prepared to let go than we were. "I will cremate her body and scatter the ashes in Georgian Bay, where we spent every summer. Yes, I'm ready. You can turn everything off."

I was in awe of her, her love and her ability to let go. I thought about what I should do.

"Are you telling me that a mother has to wait for a doctor to discharge his legal duty before her daughter can die?" she said in disbelief, trying to reconcile with a situation that confounded her. "What about organ donation? Can Cat donate her organs? She would have wanted that."

Her huge generosity of spirit at a time like this was astounding, but we were entering tricky and uncharted waters. Brain death was the criterion for organ donation, not cardiac death and technically speaking, Catherine's brain was not completely dead. She still took the occasional breaths, there was a flicker of a primitive reflex in her limbs. Yes, Catherine was surely dead, if not for the life support she was on, but she was not legally or medically brain-dead. "You can donate her tissues and bones after the machines are turned off," I explained, "but not her organs."

I called the staff doctor at home. Indeed, why should she have to wait if this was her belief in the face of incontrovertible medical facts that were documented and not in dispute? He agreed with me and regretted the fact that she did not qualify to be an organ donor. We could sympathize with how donating her daughter's organs could bring some redemption to an otherwise inexplicable, tragic event, but it was legally unprecedented. I returned to the mother and sat with her as she meditated or perhaps prayed. When she indicated to me that she was ready, I got up and turned off each machine, pump, and monitor, one by one, until there was silence.

AT HOME, in my spare time, I was busy making my own quilts. Lots of colourful, slapdash, mismatched, imperfect ones made from bits and pieces of flannel baby blankets (precious stains long washed out), bits of souvenir T-shirts and cut up pieces of my husband's shirts* sewed into the mix. One night, I lay one of these quilts over my son Max as he was falling asleep. "How does that feel, sweetie?" I tucked it in all around him. "It feels like God," he said.

The nurses' quilt squares started coming in. There were the four seasons depicted in sequins and paint; dolls with different-coloured skins dressed in scrubs; a ripped apart heart sewn back together and labelled "mender of broken hearts"; a cross with appliquéd hearts in each corner; a plastic syringe filled with rhinestones, beads, gold coins, flowers, a peace sign, rainbow-coloured bits of ribbon, and candy hearts flowing out of the tip; a heart as the red, muscular organ beside one drawn as a Valentine, the symbol of love; Chinese wishes for health and good fortune in gold braid and pearlized beads; a "giving tree" with red felt hearts; nurses' hands joined to form a circle; a cat dressed up as a nurse; a cardiac rhythm strip marching across a dark night sky merging into a sunny day sky; a Hindi greeting of good wishes; curlicue Arabic script in gold glitter; embroidered words: *hope, faith, spirit, love, healing*; a caution in script: "Reckless words pierce like a sword, but the tongue of the wise brings healing. Proverbs 12:18"; Simba the Lion King and the "Circle of Life"; footprints across a starry sky; intertwined political ribbons of green, yellow, pink, and white symbolizing various causes; a plaid tartan heart from the "Maritime Nurses"; an embroidered white nursing cap with stripes on the wings; Hebrew letters inside a Star of David that spelled *refuah shlemah*, a wish for a renewal of body and spirit; a stethoscope over felt red hearts with music notes coming out of the bell,

---

* Thus, explaining the missing items from your closet, Ivan, should you happen to read this.

and a welcoming cottage with chimney and curtains at the windows.

And *hands* were all over that quilt! Hands reaching out to each other against a blue sky, white clouds as in Michelangelo's *Creation of Adam* from the Sistine Chapel; hands intertwined in a circle; a dark hand reaching out to comfort a light hand; interwoven red and purple hands, labelled "hope" and "faith," covered with sequins. Only a few nurses signed their names; most did not.

As I gazed at the quilt, I thought of all the patients who had been cared for by the hands of the nurses whose hands also created this work of art. Janet, an experienced nurse and an expert seamstress, pieced it together on her sewing machine. The quilt was finished and it was spectacular. A date was set to unveil it to the public during a dedication ceremony scheduled to take place during Nurses' Week in May 2003. But suddenly, SARS[*] broke out and the hospital was closed, all patients and many staff put under quarantine. There was a spooky, eerie feeling in the hospital, as overnight it became a ghost town. SARS brought the hospital and the entire city of Toronto to a standstill. Only essential workers, meaning nurses and some doctors, came to work. Nurses' Week was cancelled. The quilt was folded up and stored away.

Many caregivers risked their lives, quite a few got sick, and a few tragically died in the service of caring for SARS patients. Thankfully, most of us in our ICU survived intact. We learned some very hard-won, important lessons about infection control and developed a much greater appreciation of the enormity of the risks involved in caring for our patients.

Recently, quietly one afternoon, the Nurses' Comfort Quilt was mounted behind glass in the waiting room. It can be found hanging on the wall, in between the window and the fish tank.

---

[*] Severe Acute Respiratory Syndrome – a 2003 global epidemic during which thousands became ill and more than eight hundred people died.

11

A NIGHT IN THE LIFE

Sleep, nature's soft nurse.

– William Shakespeare

E ven after all these years, I still work night shifts. I probably could find a day job or an excuse to get out of them, but I'm not yet ready to say goodbye to the nights. However, on my evening drive to work along the darkening city streets, I often think about the long night ahead of me (especially about three o'clock in the morning or so, when the jokes begin to run thin or have petered out altogether and fatigue threatens to take over), and I wonder how much longer I will be able to keep this up. As I contemplate the night ahead, I dread that desperate moment that comes at least once, when I'll have to make a huge leap of faith to believe that the morning will really come.

When I go to work at night, most people I know are settling down for bedtime. I'm out of synch with my family's schedule. My "weekend" might be in the middle of the week. Friends often complain that they never know when to call me. (Do they think a nurse would allow precious sleep to be interrupted by the telephone? We unplug it or turn off the ringer!) "What's a typical shift like?" someone asked me recently and since a typical shift might just as likely be a night, I decided to keep a running log. Here goes.

Pre-Night Shift Jitters

My unease dissipates as soon as I arrive and realize once again
the hospital at night is a different place. It's more humble, no
longer bustling with self-importance as it is during the day. There
are no staff doctors and scientists in suits and white lab coats
charging around. The flurry of retail activity has ground to a halt.
You encounter far fewer lost and bewildered folks asking for
directions to the Endoscopy Suite or Radiation department. We
are workers, all of us, no managers or bosses around – all mice,
no cats – and there's a sense of solidarity in the understanding that
we will take charge in ways we wouldn't dare – nor be expected
to – during the day. To be sure, some nights are quiet and even
offer opportunities to relax. Unless, of course, someone suddenly
gets *really* sick.

1900: At the Nurses' Station

Roberta, the nurse in charge tonight, looks worried. We're short-
staffed, even with Beryl unexpectedly showing up, mistakenly
thinking she was scheduled to work. As it turns out, we need her,
"But even if we didn't, I'd keep her here for her own safety,"
Roberta mutters. We chuckle because although Beryl is a decent
nurse, a journeyman, she's not the brightest star in the sky. It's
Roberta's third night in a row, an overtime shift, and no matter
how tired she may be, or preoccupied with her personal problems
being the family's sole breadwinner (her husband died of a heart
attack a year ago), I've never seen her fatigue show, except maybe
a little bit, tonight.

(Well, at least it's not one of those change-the-clock nights at the
end of daylight saving time when we "fall back" and end up having
to work an extra hour. The union finally managed to get the hospital to pay us for that extra hour. It was only an hour, but no one
wanted to be forced to volunteer their services for free, especially
for an extra hour of night duty.)

Noreen is pacing outside her patient's door. She's the day nurse
and wants to get out in time to make it to her daughter's soccer
game. I hotfoot it over there a few minutes early to avoid her
wrath. She thanks me and launches straight into the story of the

patient we will share, back and forth, over the next few days and nights. I am listening to her as I glance across the room to Monica, my partner, who gives me a thumbs up to indicate that whatever happens, we'll deal with it and have a sweet night. "This is Mr. Lee, a sixty-eight-year-old man who came in a week ago in respiratory distress and septic shock," Noreen introduces the patient to me. "Got him off the Levophed and blood pressure remained stable . . . his temp stayed down. Extubated this afternoon . . . chest sounds clear and gases are good . . . saturations stayed in the nineties all day on forty per cent oxygen by facemask. His urine was about fifteen cc per hour, so I got an order for a diuretic." She scans the flow sheet where we make our recordings to ensure she hasn't missed any important details. "He's a *peach*, so if there's an admission during the night, he'll have to be transferred out so that you can take an arrest from the floor or a new admission from emerge. You know how it is." *I do.*

2000: Initial Assessment

I take the first hour of my shift to examine my patient and learn him organ by organ, from head to toe and inside out. He is uncommunicative, so I try to pick up his energy and sense his personality. I study his "machines" and memorize their numbers, modes, settings, and alarm limits. I lower the lights around his bed and have taken up my seat at the desk just outside the room to read the chart when Jenna, whom I had noticed earlier looking distraught, scoots out of her room, pulls up a chair beside me, and gets right to the point.

"My gynecologist – what a jerk!"

After three years of trying to get pregnant – not that she hasn't enjoyed that part of it – Jenna now wonders if it's worth it. The tests, hormone injections, the cost, and the emotional rollercoaster she's been on – maybe it's not meant to be? "At the last minute, he cancels my appointment and his secretary reschedules me for tomorrow at eleven o'clock, when I need to sleep after this night shift."

A thought occurs to me. "Have you ever considered getting off of nights for a while?" I want to ask her, but she has to hurry back to her patient before she has a chance to answer.

I've learned how to cope with practically any situation that can arise in the ICU, no matter how difficult or stressful, as long as I have a partner I can rely upon and Monica is certainly that. She is an excellent nurse, confident and competent, though bossy and judgmental at times. But Monica has a secret, wild side that not many know about. She was teased about her name during the Monica Lewinsky thing, but it didn't bother her in the least. "I would have fallen for Clinton, too," she said shamelessly. She often says she's prepared to try anything once and thankfully what she tried one year after the ICU staff Christmas party happened only once. She came to work hungover and convinced someone to start an IV and give her a litre of fluid and Gravol. She hung the IV on a coat hook in the staff lounge and lay down to sleep it off. Despite her own antics she is quick to find fault with other nurses who behave in a manner of which she disapproves. "We've got to get the lazy and overweight nurses dragonboat rowing or start a hockey team," she often says. She herself is petite, pretty, and keeps herself incredibly buff with a daily 6 a.m. spinning class at the gym. I've never seen her eat anything but carrot sticks and protein shakes and she's always throwing out the boxes of candy that families bring in to thank us and replacing them with fruit. But I admire that as a divorced single mother with a deadbeat ex-husband, working overtime and extra shifts at other hospitals, Monica has raised and supported her daughter all by herself. On top of all that, she's working toward a Master's degree in nursing administration. We all predict she'll go far.

I record my patient's vital signs, listen to his lungs, give him IV medications, a bath, back rub, and change of linen. With the assistance of Stanislaw, one of our hospital assistants, I reposition him to make him more comfortable. When I wish him a good night, I swear I can see gratitude in his eyes. When I come out of his room, Roberta is making her rounds to see how the patients are and if anyone needs help. She looks a bit tense, so I play my little game with her. "Born to Be Wild," I toss out and she calls back, "Mars Bonfire, the *Steppenwolf* album," without missing a beat. Ten years of working with her and none of us has managed to stump her yet.

The phone is ringing at the nurses' station. "Tilda, pick up line two," I hear over the intercom. It's my patient's wife, asking how he's doing. "He's fine. I've just gotten him ready to sleep." I'm pleased to tell her.

"Will he make it? Through the night, I mean?"

"Yes . . . I think so," I say cautiously. "Anything can happen, as you know, but I think he'll have a good night," I add more reassuringly. There are no guarantees, which is what I suspect she wishes I would offer. I don't mention the possibility that he may be transferred to the floor during the night if the need arises, but perhaps I should so it won't come as a surprise if it happens?

"Give him my love," she says, and I return to my patient and do just that.

2100: Time to Kick Them Out!

The overhead announcement system comes on. "Visiting hours are now over!"

"Remember that sweetie who used to be on the switchboard?" we recall fondly. "How he used to give the weather reports and advice?"

"Whatever happened to him?" someone asks, but no one knows.

Since everything is hunky-dory with my patient, I take up my post just outside his room, where I can keep an eye on everything. Hopefully, he senses I'm there and feels reassured so that he can feel safe and sleep. I sit back and sink into the quiet lull of the early night. When these interludes come, I ride their gentle wave like a dreamy lifeguard, fixing my gaze out at the ocean, scanning the horizon for trouble, always in a state of relaxed vigilance, and ready to spring into action and dive in at a moment's notice.

"What's new, Monica?" I ask when she joins me at the desk we share. She's serious about her studies, but I am aware of certain extra-curricular activities that keep her fairly busy as well.

"I do have a meeting . . . later on," she says, looking at my face to assess my reaction.

Ah, yes, I remember. "How's it going with you-know-who?" I ask, knowing perfectly well the name of the very married surgeon she's told me about.

"There's a transplant scheduled, tonight." She smiles and returns to her charting.

I connect the dots. Roberta had mentioned that an organ donor had been brought in this afternoon, brain-dead after a head-on collision. In the brief window between the harvesting of the organs and their reconnection to the recipient, there might be just enough time for a romantic tryst.

2200: To Stand or to Sit?

I wander over to the nurses' station to joke around with Roberta, but she's preoccupied. She's going over the staffing for tomorrow morning and at the same time receiving updates about a patient in the operating room who is going sour and troubleshooting problems as they come at her from all directions. All twenty-two beds are full tonight with fully ventilated, sick patients, but she's got the situation completely under control. She pauses to mention that the family of one of our patients has given us forty dollars to order pizza. "It's really decent of them, considering he's not doing very well," she says wryly.

We often enjoy wonderful meals on night shifts. Occasionally we call for a potluck and everyone brings something. It used to be pasta salads, sausage rolls, and macaroni and cheese, but over time, we have become more diverse and sophisticated. We now have Philippino noodles called *pansit*, Greek *dolmades* with lemon sauce, Indian *samosas* with tamarind chutney, and Jamaican *rotis*. Tonight, I see only a dismal bag of stale jujubes on the desk, but Oscar, a nurse originally from Guyana, tells us he has brought in a big pot of "cook-up" – a rice dish. "It's in the staff lounge, help yourselves," he says. "But it may be too spicy for you Joneses and Smiths," he warns with a grin.

We've celebrated many birthdays, weddings, and baby showers together. There are always notices plastered all around the walls of the ICU, and not just for these social events, but also for workshops, conferences, or information about new tools and technology. There are always a few posted on the inside of the door in each bathroom. Presumably, they are placed there because the majority of the readers are female and, therefore, face the door. I postulate that gender equality will have been achieved in nursing when there are an equal number of notices on the wall behind the toilet seat as there are facing the toilet!

2210: A Critical Call

Someone, somewhere is very sick and needs to come to us. "How are we for beds?" I assume the resident is asking Roberta on the phone because she answers, "Beds? Plenty of 'em! It's nurses we're short of." She rolls her eyes and covers the receiver. "Why don't people get this? We need more nurses, not furniture." Roberta looks at the list of patients' names and the list of nurses' names and thinks out loud. "I'll have to double up two patients, prepare the rooms for the liver and a lung transplant coming out of the OR, and move a few people around, but it sounds like this patient needs to come here." She hangs up the phone and I follow after her to give her a hand preparing the room for the new admission. "At least you won't have to be on standby to transfer your patient out after all, Tilda," Roberta says.

"How so?" I had just been regretting that I hadn't warned the wife that might happen.

"Casey's patient just died, so she's free to take this new patient." Roberta flips on the overhead light and the cardiac monitor, which emits a humming, then a buzzing, as if it, too, is gearing up for the action ahead. She goes out into the hall to stop Tariq, the respiratory therapist, to let him know that a patient is on the way. "She's a twenty-five-year-old, found unconscious at home, with an empty bottle of Tylenol beside her. She'll be here in a few hours by helicopter from Sudbury," she tells him so that he can get a ventilator ready. "Yes, Casey will admit her," she explains to me, "as soon as she finishes her arts and crafts project, or whatever it is she's doing." Roberta waves at Casey, who's sitting at the nurses' station, busy with yards of bright pink fabric. I stop to ask Casey what she's up to and pull out yards of silky fabric from her huge shopping bag. There's a salami sandwich in there, too, I see. Until her patient arrives, she's working on a bridesmaid's dress she's making for a friend's wedding.

Around 2300, or So: A Messy Situation[*]

Trina needs our help. In preparation, we don gowns, masks, vinyl gloves and with Jenna and I on one side of the bed, we roll the patient toward us. Trina is on the other side with a pile of wet, warm washcloths ready to get to work. It started with a few dabs, then a smear. Now, it's a slow ooze.

"That's it! I'll never be able to eat chocolate pudding again," Jenna whispers and looks away.

Shhh, we say, suppressing our own equally unsavoury, naughty, uncharitable, unprofessional thoughts. *Thank goodness the patient is unconscious!*

Now it's morphing from dark squirts to bubbly ribbons. It's flowing, gathering speed. I hand Trina more wet washcloths and picture the little Dutch boy with his finger in the dyke to stem the flood. I cough a little to expel the smell. Stay focused on the patient, not the smell or the sight, Frances used to say to me. It's advice that actually helps. "You're doing fine," I whisper into the patient's ear, whether he can hear me or not.

Now it's a river, pouring out faster than Trina can wipe it away. *Rollin', rollin', rollin',* . . . We stand there, waiting it out while it streams down the patient's legs, into the folds of his scrotum, around his catheter. Our gloves are slippery and there are now flecks and streaks on the front and sleeves of our gowns. It's a force of nature, like lava pouring forth still smouldering from inside a human cave.

This experience is no longer what it was for me in the past, but I had to overcome my own shame before I could help patients deal with theirs. I do not consider this work demeaning or degrading. It is not humiliating, disgusting, or repulsive. It is not boring or tedious or anxiety-provoking. I accept it. It is what it is. It's life itself. It's an opportunity to help restore dignity and I do it with as much finesse as I can. I put my hand on the patient's shoulder. "It's okay," I say.

It has taken me such a long time to get here.

---

[*] Please note: The following would be a good passage to read if you are trying to lose weight. It may be an effective appetite suppressant.

We stay until the flow abates sufficiently for Trina to put the finishing touches on the job by herself and we hustle out of the room. We strip off our gowns and gloves and gather at the sinks and now that we are sufficiently out-of-range and "offstage," we let loose, a little.

"That was a *poo-nami*!" Jenna says, laughing helplessly. "It reminds me of the time a patient shit on my head," she says. "I'll never forget it. It was purely accidental, of course, but I was leaning down to tuck in the sheets and out it came, spurt, spurt, spurt, all over me. Liquid poo was dripping down my bangs and forehead. I ran out and hosed myself down."

"Why do so many of our patients have diarrhea?" I muse. "Is it from the antibiotics? The feeds? The stress?" (Note to self: Do an online search of diarrhea-related scientific literature.)

"What about my invention?" Theo comes over to tell us. "Before giving the patient a bedpan," he explains, "first, line it with an incontinence pad. That makes it warm and cozy for the patient's bum and afterward, voilà, you wrap up the entire bagatelle, that splendid little package, and dispose pronto. No rinsing or scraping. No spraying and having back splash comin' at ya! Make sure you prepare another one all ready for the next event!"

"That is life-changing advice, Theo," I say solemnly, sincerely.

At 2359: Just Before Midnight

Monica's gone on her break. I check on the patients and then dash out to get some supplies. On the way back I run into Jenna, who looks worried and I'm fairly certain it's not about her ovulation cycle. "Take a look at this." She hands me a clipboard upon which her patient has written a note to her. "Ever since I lightened his sedation he's been frantically trying to tell me something."

It's a wobbly scrawl, but we make out "daughter" and "alone." Jenna's patient has pneumonia related to HIV he got from sharing needles. "I asked how old his daughter is and I'm pretty sure he held up six fingers." Jenna looks worried. "Do you think he's trying to tell me she's been left alone?"

Roberta comes over, flipping through the chart for clues. "He was brought in by ambulance to emerge. No one came with him.

There's nothing in the chart." She sighs. "They could look into it on the day shift," she thinks aloud, "but on the other hand, it might be urgent. I'll call the police and ask them to check into it," she decides and hurries off.

0000: The Missing Minute

Midnight is 0000 hours in our digital world. Is it the end of the night or the beginning of the next day? Is it today's date or tomorrow's? So far, this night is allowing me to consider such imponderables. I listen in on Roberta talking to a family member at home. She's trying to soften the blow after the doctor called to tell them their eighty-four-year-old father died. (It's not in her to fabricate by telling people their loved one has "taken a turn for the worse," even if they have just died so that they won't drive crazy on the way in like many well-meaning nurses do.) That must have been Casey's patient, I figure. He had an abdominal aneurysm and was scheduled for surgery the very next day, but the family doesn't seem shocked by the news. Roberta offers them the opportunity to come see the body, but they decline. "I'm sorry for your loss," she says.

0033: The Tools of Our Trade

I get up to stretch my legs and set off, on the prowl for something sweet or salty to nibble on, out of a vague restlessness. I see the nightly congregation about the nurses' station has begun. We're a few steps away from our patients' rooms and can be there in a jiffy if needed, but for a few moments it is as if we are a world away. It's our communal campfire and there's no denying that at times, there's a festive, party atmosphere that must seem so heartless to anyone passing by. Here we sit with our jellybeans and pretzels and over there are the patients, stretched out with their tube feedings and IV bags. We are chatting and laughing while they are intubated and unconscious. Not for one moment are we oblivious to the fact that they are not exactly having quite as merry a time as we are, but somehow, that brief, frivolous interlude fortifies us to return to our patients. Perhaps at times we do get carried away. I remember a patient on the floor telling me once, "I heard you guys and dolls whoopin' it up last night. Having a party, were you?" I apologized for keeping him up. "Yeah, but it was also kinda nice hearing your young voices and knowing at least someone is having a good time," he admitted.

Tonight we're worrying about our hands, the tools of our trade. We examine them for cuts, abrasions, contact dermatitis, and rashes. We bemoan the antimicrobial hand lotion we have to constantly use, and how it dries the skin.

"It's the powder inside the gloves that irritates them, makes them itchy."

"My hands are raw! Worse on the days I work and on my days off, they kind of recover."

"All the handwashing we do is rough on the skin."

"I can't stand wearing gloves. It's not the same, you know, when you touch a patient through vinyl. It's like wearing a . . ."

"Yes, yes, we know, we get it."

We moisturize. We debate the merits of glycerine, lanolin, shea butter, and plain old Vaseline. We vote for the most effective barrier cream, the best emollient, and estimate the number of hand scrubs per shift. We keep our hands in good shape, the way a chef cares for his set of knives or a musician tunes his instrument. We were impressed when we heard about a hospital that gave out leather manicure kits for Nurses' Week – much preferable to the coffee mugs with the hospital's logo, pizza vouchers, or free doughnuts, we all agreed.

I greet Chandra, who's also on tonight. She's dipping her fingers into an industrial-sized pot of something called "Bag Balm," working it into her hands. It smells like a barnyard. "Have you seen what it says here?" I read the label. "For veterinary use only. It's a 'soothing, penetrating, healing ointment for caked bags, sore teats, and chapped, hard milkers. Apply to udders before the night milking and again before the day milking.'"

"If it's good enough for Shania Twain, it's good enough for me."

"She uses it? What's wrong with *her* hands?"

I put to them a question I'd been thinking about. "Could you be a nurse if you were blind?" They ponder a moment then mostly agree. Even in a wheelchair, you could be a nurse, they say. "But what if you didn't have use of your hands?" Ahh, that's different, they agree. No, without hands, you couldn't be a nurse.

"That's what I think. No gadget, device, piece of equipment, or trained monkeys will ever replace the hardworking human hand, for its capacity to soothe," I say, bringing them around to my foregone conclusion.

Roberta makes like she's playing the violin to my sentimental observations.

"Oh, cry me a river!" says Jenna.

Theo joins us and we admire his beautiful hands and the elegant gold and sapphire band he's been wearing on his ring finger since his recent wedding to his partner, Phillip. "Boop-boop-dee-boop," he sings out, giving a little skip and kick of his heels before plopping himself down onto Roberta's lap. He has shown me pictures of when he was a drag queen and won the Ms. Gay Halifax Pageant and, I must say, he looked stunning in his pale blue ball gown.

At the start of every shift, Theo swoops into the ICU and envelops each person he encounters into a huge embrace and plants a kiss on every cheek of each doctor, nurse, hospital assistant, porter, housekeeper, respiratory therapist, ward clerk, family member. "I darn near got a hernia leaning into your bed to give you that kiss," I once heard him say to a patient. No one is left unhugged or unkissed by Theo, whether they like it or not, and most everyone does. (And if at first they aren't completely comfortable with such florid demonstrations of affection, they soon get used to it and even begin to crave it.)

I've often wondered why there aren't more men in nursing. Back when I graduated in 1983 about 2 per cent of nurses were male. Nowadays, they say it's about 5 per cent – not much progress toward gender balance. I have worked with only a few dozen men over the years, most of them decidedly straight, quite a few openly gay, one (that I knew of) who was transgendered, and a few undecided – but who cares? What difference does it make? What is really mind-boggling is that there are not more men in nursing, still in 2007. I once asked Theo how he chose nursing.

"It drove my father crazy when I told him," he said, "but I think he's come around. I've always known I wanted to be a nurse. The guidance counsellor at school spent two hours one day trying to get me to change my mind. He said, 'Theo, what about medicine or law?' But I didn't want to be a doctor and I knew I wasn't a good enough liar to be a lawyer!"

"Why aren't there more men in nursing, Theo?"

"It's different for gay men. We don't feel we have to hide our soft, caring side, but most straight guys are afraid it will make people raise questions about their sexuality."

I can feel my own soft, caring side beginning to flag at this time of the night, so I ask Roberta to recite one of her latest poems to perk us all up. Not many know that in addition to her vast store of rock 'n' roll trivia, Roberta has another talent. She is secretly a poet. "I tossed this one off this morning, before going to sleep." She pulls a sheet of paper from her pocket. "It's called 'Just One Shock.'"

> I need to see the doctor
> I need to hear the news
> I only want the good stuff
> Don't be giving me the blues
>
> I'll ask one hundred questions
> Then I'll ask one hundred more, but
> If you don't give me good news,
> Then I'm heading for the door.
>
> As soon as you start saying
> That he will not pull through
> That's the time that I will say
> Don't call me, I'll call you
>
> Let me make this clear to you
> Before I get to my car
> I want you to do everything
> I've seen it on *ER*
>
> He's only eighty-eight, you see
> Enough of all this talk
> If his heart should stop tonight
> I expect you to give one more shock.

How true, we murmured, appreciatively. *At least someone has the guts to tell it like it is.*

Theo gets up and stretches his arms over his head. "Tootle-loo, chums. See ya, later."

Chandra returns to her patient so that her partner, Tikki, can get away for a break and Jenna has already left. She seems in a much cheerier mood since her pager went off a few minutes ago and she showed me the text message from her husband, who is a policeman, also working the night shift. "I . . . LOVE . . . YOU," the digital letters spelled out. I don't think I've ever seen anything more romantic.

I stay behind with Roberta, who is quiet. She has told me about her latest family worry. In addition to one son with autism, her other son was just diagnosed with Tourette's Syndrome. "I used to call us the A-team, but I guess now, we'll be the 'T and A' team," she says.

I want to tell her again that I admire how she deals with her challenges, but it makes her cringe whenever I do. "You gotta do what you gotta do. You'd do the same if you had to," she's told me. "It's like being a nurse. You don't want to be thought of as a hero or an angel. You're an ordinary person doing a difficult job with good days and bad days." She gets up to make her rounds, but before she goes, I can't resist.

"Life Is a Highway," I sing out to her.

"Tom Cochrane, and I'm going to be driving it for a long while," she sighs.

Trina flies past us at the nurses' station. "Yo, you vanilla girls, get your butts in my room," she, a chocolate girl, says. "I need your muscles to turn my patient and change the sheets again."

Roberta goes to help her and I return to my own patient. It's about time I got back to work.

0100: Priority Setting

When time permits and all is quiet, we take turns and steal away for a break. Jenna is carrying a blanket, in search of a place to nap. "That one is haunted," she says, rejecting a particular room.

"There's a ghost. Remember that young boy who died? Well, I'm not going in there," she says, superstition overriding her fatigue.

I pay a short visit to Tikki, ostensibly to say hello, but my hidden agenda is to check up on her and she knows it. When she started in the ICU a few months ago, I was her preceptor. She came to us straight from her university studies where she achieved top marks. She's now qualified to "fly solo," but a few of us have an uneasy feeling about her and I always try to be nearby, especially if she has a really *busy* patient. There is no question that Tikki has improved, but to be honest, the thing that changes most noticeably about her is her hair. She started out with a spiky, black Goth style to a fancy up-do with purple streaks, to her current style of long, multi-coloured dreadlocks. In addition to her many tattoos she's shown us, she's got lots of body piercings – tongue and ears are what's visible, but she claims there's more. (Funny, I saw her once with her mother in the supermarket wearing a girly, puffy ski jacket and a lavender Dora the Explorer track suit. Go figure.) She's now a Wiccan and a devotee of hypnotic techno music. She has a new tattoo she wants to show me and informs me that her diamond nose ring is actually an engagement ring. I'm just about to offer congratulations when I notice two long cords dangling from her ears, snaking into her scrubs. *She's listening to music?* "Tikki, is that an iPod?" I am aghast. She is moving to the beat of the music in her ears and doesn't hear me so I tug on one of the strings. "Tikki, you won't hear the alarms! You can't concentrate properly!" I stop. There are more reasons than I could possibly enumerate. "Take it off!"

"Hey, Tikki can you give me a hand with my patient's dressing change?" Chandra, on the other side of the room, calls out to her.

"I'll be there in a minute. I have a bid on eBay in five minutes for a vintage Barbie, okay?"

Chandra and I lock eyes in irritation. "No, Tikki, it's not okay. I need your help now." Tikki turns off her music and logs off her computer.

I quell the terrible feeling I have at what I have just seen and return to my own patient. I sit at the desk and open a file in which I've been making notes and collecting data for the past few weeks. I add Tikki's newest tattoo. It's a green-blue serpent on her ankle. I keep watch over my patient and review my findings.

0115: Home Alone

It seems Jenna's patient's six-year-old daughter was indeed left alone when her father suddenly took ill and was brought to the Emergency department. Fortunately, a neighbour took her in and she's being cared for by Children's Aid Services until her father gets back on his feet. How easily Jenna and Roberta could have let that go, passed the buck, or overlooked it altogether. How easily they could have said, I'm tired, or it's not my concern, it's beyond our scope. "Good call, Roberta," I say, but she shrugs it off.

"Good friends, neighbours – isn't that what people need more than anything?"

"Tonight's the Night," I put to her.

"Rod Stewart. Hey, what research are you up to?" She pointed at my stack of notes and I smile an inscrutable smile. "You're So Vain," I tease her with Carly Simon.

0130: Research That Gets Under Their Skin

Of thirty-eight subjects, between the ages of twenty-five and fifty-five, including nurses, respiratory therapists, doctors, and one hospital attendant, 68 per cent have at least one tattoo. Here is a representative sampling:

A dolphin on a hip, a ring of roses around an ankle, Woody Woodpecker on an inner thigh, a green Celtic symbol behind an ear; a Brazilian wax,[*] numerous butterflies, the names Tom and Terry, a Toronto Maple Leafs logo; yin and yang; the Mona Lisa, a marijuana leaf, and an @ sign, a dragon, a cross, a Nike swoosh (the ultimate branding), a sword, Chinese characters, and a skull and crossbones.

And some noteworthy narrative comments:

---

[*] Though not a tattoo, still noteworthy body art in its own right.

An obstetrician passing by, eager to be included in my "study," told me about her first delivery. "I lifted the patient's gown and right there, on her pubic area, was . . ." She stopped to laugh at the memory, "Tweety-Bird! Well, what could I say but, 'I tot I taw a puddy-tat?' The staff doc bent down to take a look and he's normally a very uptight sort of guy, but he said with a perfectly straight face, 'I did, I did! I did see a puddy-tat!'"

A hospital attendant reported that he once worked in a tattoo parlour. "It was near a church and you wouldn't believe how many priests – and nuns, too – came in to have religious symbols – as well as some kinkier things – put on under their clothes where they'll never be seen."

Only one day by your nurse, I thought. *We'll see everything.*

0140: No Rest for the Weary

"Have You Lost That Lovin' Feelin'?" I ask Roberta as she rushes past me.

"No! The Righteous Brothers. What makes you think that?"

"Having any 'Saturday Night Fever'?" I ask her, pretending to be concerned.

"The Brothers Gibb," she says without pausing. "I'm busy. I've got to help Casey admit the new patient." Casey has indeed put aside her sewing and salami and is back to her usual efficient and capable self, busy with the young woman who overdosed on Tylenol and her distraught parents. I go over to help, but as chaotic as it is in there, Casey has everything under control. The room is filled with lots of doctors, nurses, and respiratory therapists, and they don't need another pair of hands, so I head back to my patient. I can't help but remember similar situations in the past with Laura, who would be right in the midst of this crisis, taking control of the emergency, but afterward felt compelled to make some caustic remark like, "I'm going to give a seminar called, 'Suicide: Get It Right the First Time.'" Laura had a problem with these patients. "They botch themselves up and make life worse,"

she'd pretend to complain, for she couldn't reconcile that we were
fighting to save lives and they were trying to destroy theirs, but as
usual, expressed her sadness as outrage.

A chaplain, looking just as distraught as the family, stands
outside the patient's room, consoling them. The mother, through
her sobs, tells the doctor and Casey what happened. "She had a
terrible fight with her boyfriend. He was cheating on her and she
went home and swallowed a bottle of Tylenol, chased down with
alcohol. There was no note."

I shiver, suddenly feeling cold, and return to my patient's room,
where I'm supposed to be, anyway. It's not my particular assigned
portion of tragedy tonight.

0150 or So: Low Tide

No matter how many years of working nights, I still feel a chill
and an overwhelming urge to lie down about now. Night shift
doesn't feel healthy. It's not normal and it's getting harder as I get
older. You don't sleep the same way during the day as you do at
night. How much longer can I keep this up? From time to time,
someone brings in an article about higher rates of migraines,
depression, breast cancer, stomach problems, infertility, and heart
disease in night shift workers. We worry. I make a list of things I've
got to do on my day off. It's time for the second wind to kick in.
Where is it?

0200: Vampires

We move from bed to bed, drawing samples of blood from our
patients' arteries and veins. We need some results right away to
treat any abnormal values and others to have ready to review by
morning rounds. Luckily, we don't have to wake our patients and
can do it silently, drawing our samples from lines already in place.
Bone-weary, cement-footed, dragged down, my vision is blurred,
my mind is foggy, and my thoughts are muddled. *I'm getting too
old for this.* I get up and walk around, splash cold water on my
face at the sink. I will myself awake with whatever mental powers
I can summon. The second wind must be right around the corner,

any minute now it'll come. How short the night feels when you're sleeping in your bed at home and how long it feels when you are up all night at work. I skulk around the unit, eavesdropping, guarding, gossiping, and watching.

0300: The Witching Hour

Three o'clock in the morning feels like the middle of the night, but there are only four more hours to go. Monica has returned from her "break," looking flushed and more energized than anyone has a right to at this hour of the night. She is shocked when I tell her about Tikki's iPod and bad attitude and asks me what I am going to do about it. She tells me I'd better keep my eye on her and document the problems with her work. "If you see something wrong, it's your duty to do something about it," she reminds me and I know she's right.

Tikki is not too pleased when I show at her side once again. I hate policing people, but when I take one look at her patient's flow sheet, I immediately see a problem that could be serious. "Tikki, did you notice your patient's cardiac output?"

"Yes, I did," she says slowly. "It's 2.3 litres per minute."

"What did you do about it?"

"I mentioned to the doctor it was low," Tikki said defensively, "but she didn't react."

"You have to recognize the significance, make a fuss, and follow through," I say, trying to goad some reaction out of her, but she only looks wounded and starts to explain herself. Suddenly, across the room, there's a scream and a moan.

"Help! I need help!"

It's Chandra. I leap over in two bounds. In moments, Roberta rushes in. Theo arrives, pushing the crash cart ahead of him, Jenna, Trina, and others right behind him. Chandra is slumped over the side rails of her patient's bed, practically lying on top of her patient, her hands covering her face. "Shit, shit. I've made a terrible mistake." She pulls herself upright and quells her terror long enough to tell us exactly what happened. "I hung what I thought was the antibiotic, but it was a bag of insulin – fifty units in a fifty cc bag. I got them mixed up. Instead of the antibiotic, I ran in the entire bag of insulin in twenty minutes. It was supposed to go in over twenty-four hours."

She's barely finished getting this story out and Roberta has already run to fetch the glucose analyzer to check the blood sugar and I am pushing two large syringes of Dextrose 50 per cent – D50 – a concentrated sugar solution, into the patient's central intravenous line. Someone pages the doctor. We work fast. Chandra is in shock, stunned by what she's done. Normally a self-possessed, take-charge sort of person who prefers to do everything herself, she's backed right off and lets us take over, as if she's forfeited her right to be a nurse.

Theo examines the patient, assessing his level of consciousness. He shines a light into his eyes and sees that the pupils are responding briskly, as they should. Someone draws blood to check electrolytes. As I place the electrodes on the patient's limbs and chest for a twelve-lead ECG, I catch sight of Tikki, watching and looking smug. Surely she recognizes that this is an emergency? "He looks okay to me," she says with a shrug of her shoulders and goes back to her own work.

"He may not be shortly," I snap at her, glancing at the blood sugar result of 3.0 mmol/L.* Anything below 4.0 is dangerously low. *Don't you realize if we don't take immediate action to rescue him, he will have a seizure, go into a coma, and have a cardiac arrest in a matter of minutes?* I draw up a syringe of midazolam, the treatment for a sudden seizure, to have at the ready. The patient stirs in his sleep and we jump. Is it due to the commotion in the room or the sudden plummeting of blood sugar? Theo tries to shake him awake, but can't rouse him. Whether it's from insulin shock or from the sedation he's already on, we can't tell. I push in another – now the third ampoule of D50 and Roberta retests the patient's blood sugar. It's now 2.5 and could still drop further. "Is the doctor on her way?" I ask.

"She can't come right now," Roberta says. She's starting a Dextrose 10 per cent solution and I push in another amp of D50,

---

* International Units.

figuring that even if I overshoot, a high sugar level is less danger-ous than a low one, and set my eyes on the cardiac monitor, on the lookout for arrhythmias. "She's in emerge examining a patient who may have to come here and the young woman with the Tylenol overdose is crashing, so she has to go to her first, but she says we're doing all the correct things."

"How could I be so stupid?" Chandra moans. She paces the room, wringing her hands. "I wasn't tired. I wasn't overly busy. I wasn't stressed out." She stops in front of the IV pump, picks up the empty bag of insulin in her hand, stares at it, and shakes her head as she searches for clues to understand her mistake. I can imagine her desperate wish to take back those few moments of in-attention, to return to the blissful, innocent time of "just before."

"He'll be okay," I say, taking another reading, and see that the blood sugar is down to 1.6. I push in two more amps of D50. *I think he will, anyway.*

0400: The Correction

We've managed to get the patient's blood sugar back to a normal range and so far, he does not seem to be experiencing any adverse effects from the mistake. I put my arm around Chandra, who is devastated. She pulls away and I understand her reaction. What I do not understand is Tikki's.

The doctor arrives and says, "You saved her," and doesn't harp on the fact that one of us almost killed her. She is pleased we took control and agrees with everything we've done. She examines the patient, finds no abnormalities, and is satisfied that the mistake has been completely rectified. She and Chandra fill in an incident report that outlines all the details. In the morning, they will inform the manager and staff doctor, who will call the family to let them know what happened.

We all can see how hard it is for Chandra and we realize she wants space. She has retreated inward and is inaccessible. She's lost trust in herself as a nurse. She's trying to find her way back, learning to be a nurse all over again. She pulls away from us as if this self-imposed isolation is part of her punishment.

0500: On Guard

Who needs a "second wind" now? There's nothing like a crisis like that to jolt me out of my fatigue! I return to my patient's room and stand at the window to catch my breath, one eye, as always, on the monitor. It is quiet in the room, other than the bubble and hiss of his oxygen set-up. I look out at the city from the top of University Avenue, right down to Lake Ontario. I am rattled not only by the mistake and the nearness of fatality, but by Tikki's nonchalance. What concerns me the most was that she was not concerned in the least. Her defence was that it wasn't her patient. "They're all our patients," I said, "we work as a team." *Why do I have to tell you this?* I wanted to scream at her.

The city sleeps. My patient sleeps. I note that his hourly urine has picked up from the diuretic that Noreen had given on days and that his cardiac filling pressures have also improved. His chest sounds clear and his vital signs are normal. He's getting better.

A flashing blue light from the helicopter on the landing pad at the Hospital for Sick Children across the street flickers on the wall of my patient's room. It was the aircraft that brought in the young woman that Casey is taking care of down the hall and it's now preparing to take off to another emergency somewhere in the province. I have that nagging feeling I've had so often throughout my life, that I'm a lone, silent guardian and that it's all up to me to take care of everything. But how silly, of course I am not alone. I am a member of a team.

0600: Almost There

"Hey, Tilda," Roberta says, "do me a favour. Go check on the chaplain. I think he may be having a meltdown."

I find him sitting outside the patient's room, staring into space. As soon as I touch his shoulder, he bursts into tears. He apologizes and says he has encountered this sort of tragedy before, of course, but for some reason this one is really hitting him hard, perhaps because his own daughter is the same age as this young girl? He looks exhausted and seems traumatized. He probably should "debrief" but right now he needs to rest. I take him to a couch in the waiting room and cover him with a pile of blankets. He's shivering and grateful.

0700: Morning Has Broken

I read somewhere that the noise during shift change is as many decibels as a chainsaw. The team is arriving for the day shift and the nurses' chatter and laughter may be annoying to patients, but to us night nurses, it's the sound of salvation. We're miners, deep down in the pit, hearing sounds of life from above. Rescue is on its way! (One does tend to get a bit dramatic when sleep-deprived.) The clean, fresh nurses start bopping in, energetic and vibrant, some smelling of shampoo, their hair still damp from their morning showers. We're grubby and crabby and feel like hags and ogres. "Busy night?" the fired-up new ones ask us, graciously showing sympathy despite their sleep-saturated superiority.

"It was . . ." we look at each other to arrive at a consensus, "steady," we concur.

After handover, we sign off our charts with "Report given," and thus, relieved of our duties, we head off to the locker room where we dump our uniforms into the hospital laundry, change into our real clothes, and file out the door. We can't wait to get home and take showers. Chandra is staying behind to report her medication error to the staff doctor and Jenna goes off to the cafeteria to drink coffee and eat pancakes to keep herself awake for her gynecologist's appointment later in the morning, but the rest of us head off to the elevator. We give each other a quick once-over to check if anyone looks too bleary-eyed to drive home.[*]

We push out the door and plunge into the cool morning air, breathing deeply. Somehow, even the pollution and city smog smell fresher than the recycled hospital air we've been breathing all night. If the sky is overcast or if it's raining, we congratulate ourselves on the good sleeping conditions, but if the sun is boldly

---

[*] More times than I like to recall, I've had to pull over to the side of the road for a rest before continuing home. Once, I think I was actually sleeping while driving, but I'm not sure.

shining, mocking our upside-down lives, we moan about the beautiful day we have to waste by sleeping. We go our separate ways,
calling out "good night" to one another.

I zip along the streets, happy to be going in the opposite direction to the flow of downtown traffic. I'm ready to get into bed as
soon as I get home, but there have been many mornings after a
night shift when I've been too buzzed to go straight to sleep. Many
nurses tell me they have insomnia and have to hang heavy curtains
on their windows to keep out the blazing sun and wear earplugs
to muffle the noise of construction, traffic, doorbells, and barking
dogs. Not me, I can sleep under any conditions. But I do linger a
few minutes longer, enjoying the quiet and having the house to
myself, before crawling into bed, joined only by Digit, our six-toed
calico cat who perhaps understands best, as she is nocturnal, too.

12

NIGHTMARES

Harming a patient is every nurse's worst nightmare. Nurses know that even giving the correct medication at the wrong time, or missing a single dose of a drug is an error. If a doctor writes an order that is incorrect in any way and the nurse gives the drug as ordered, the nurse has also committed an error. Every nurse I know does everything possible to give safe care, but if I knew a nurse who was unsafe, I'd be just as wrong if I didn't do something about it. We've all made mistakes, fortunately most of them not as serious as Chandra's accidental insulin overdose. That problem was corrected, there were no consequences to the patient, and although the family was understandably upset, they accepted the apology offered. But since then, Chandra has been off work and has told me privately that she has decided to leave the ICU. Her confidence has been thoroughly shaken.

That night I realized I had my own nightmare waiting to happen: Tikki. When I saw her stand by in the aftermath of Chandra's potentially fatal error and not rush to assist her nor appear to comprehend its serious implications for the patient, I realized that Tikki was not a safe nurse. As her preceptor to the ICU, it was incumbent upon me to do something about her, and fast.

Tikki was intelligent and skilful, but did not show good judgment. Another problem was her attitude. She was cocky and fearless: she didn't know what she didn't know and not being aware of deficiencies in your knowledge is a dangerous thing in a nurse. You have to have a degree of caution, the ability to recognize subtle changes and pick up on warning signals, and ask lots of questions. You have to keep an active sense of wonder and not jump to conclusions. You have to have a sense of fear and awe and if you don't feel that edge, that's a serious problem. Tikki had way more confidence than she deserved. She never paused to consider, think things through, or question herself; she just plunged right into situations. I once saw her inject a medication through a patient's naso-gastric feeding tube without ensuring beforehand that it was positioned correctly in the patient's stomach.

"No worries," she said blithely when I mentioned it to her.

"It might have been too high up or in the trachea and the patient could have aspirated into his lungs. You have to always check it first."

She verified that the tube was in fact in the correct position. "See, it was fine all along," she said. "You were worried for nothing."

I wasn't the only one who had become uneasy about her.

"Why are you still sitting on this?" Monica took me aside on the next shift we worked together after the night of Chandra's insulin error. "Are you documenting the problems? Have you spoken to our manager? Are you on top of this, Tilda?" She was about to launch into her own litany of complaints against Tikki's nursing care, but I stopped her. I had enough evidence of my own. The question was, what was I going to do about it? She had only been working in the ICU for a short time and I had wanted to give her sufficient time to adjust and prove herself. But after that night, I realized that by doing nothing, I might be allowing something terrible to happen.

The next day we worked together, I told Tikki she had to continue to work under my supervision. There were more skills that I needed to observe her perform, I told her. I had concerns about her nursing care. She scowled. Throughout that day she pretended to listen when I pointed out problems, but then I saw her roll her eyes or ridicule me to her friends. The next shift, when she saw we were still paired, she objected. "When will I be able to be on my own? I've worked in the ICU for four months."

"You've never taken care of a patient with a chest tube," I said, mentioning the very least of my concerns.

"I did once in the computer simulation lab at university."

"But never a real patient," I pointed out. What I wanted to add but wasn't ready was a growing list of concerns: *You didn't reposition your patient for more than three hours until I told you to do so. You habitually leave your patients in soiled sheets, likely because you consider cleaning bums beneath a nurse with a university degree. You didn't check your patient's potassium level before giving him Digoxin* * *and you couldn't tell me why your patient, who was in atrial fibrillation, was also on anticoagulation medication.*† Those were just three more damning indictments of her nursing care that sprang to mind. The rest of that day went well, but at the end of the shift, I told Tikki we needed to meet to discuss some of the problems I was seeing in her practice and that I planned to speak with our manager about it.

"Whatever," she said with feigned disinterest. "But our little pow-wow will have to wait," she added with a smirk. "I'm on vacation for two weeks. I'm off to Europe for the street music festivals."

"Have a good time," I said. "Let's meet as soon as you get back."

Meanwhile, there was a buzz in the ICU about Jenna. She had also been off work for more than a month. She wasn't returning our calls and many of us were worried about her. I was more worried than the others because I knew the reason for her absence. She had called me and told me she was undergoing

---

* Serum potassium level must be within normal range before administering Digoxin to avoid arrhythmias.

† Anticoagulation therapy (blood thinners) is instituted for atrial fibrillation (a serious arrhythmia) to prevent clot formation, which can lead to a stroke.

intensive treatment for infertility that required daily visits to the
doctor and asked me to tell the others that that was the reason
she was off work. What she confided in me alone was that she
was also off work due to emotional stress.

She was in trouble with the College of Nurses, our licensing
body. A serious complaint had been lodged against her by the
family of a patient she had cared for in the ICU, more than a year
ago. They had many charges against her, but it all added up to the
accusation that Jenna's actions had led to the death of their mother.
I asked Jenna if she wanted to meet with me to talk things over
and she eagerly agreed. I wanted to reach out to a colleague in
trouble, but to be honest I also wanted to understand how this
came about in order to make sure it never happened to me. If
this nightmare could happen to a decent, competent nurse like
Jenna, it could happen to any of us.

From what I knew of Jenna, it was impossible to imagine that
she would do something purposely dangerous or harmful to a
patient. It was also hard to believe that if she had made an error,
such as Chandra had, that she would not have disclosed it. Had
she actually made a mistake, I wondered, or was there a *percep-
tion* by the family of negligence? Indeed, if Jenna was being *falsely*
accused, it's a terrible experience but it is only a nurse's *second*
worst nightmare. The first worst nightmare is to be *rightly*
accused. At any rate, I vowed to stay open-minded until I heard
all the facts from Jenna and saw the documents of the case that
she was prepared to show me. We set a date to meet.

I couldn't help but think about some of the slips, the near misses,
and mix-ups I've made or seen over the years. Fortunately, the vast
majority of them have never caused any real harm and for me only
served as useful prods to ever more attention and vigilance. But I
don't know a nurse who doesn't have a war story or two.

In the privacy of our homes, many of us practise a rather macabre
habit. As soon as we receive our bimonthly bulletin from the College
of Nurses, we tear straight to its back pages to read the accounts of
complaints lodged against nurses by members of the public,
including the explicit details of their alleged – or sometimes proven
– misdemeanours. The situations are painful to read, sobering,

shocking, flabbergasting, embarrassing, and, occasionally, mildly amusing. Thankfully, they are very rare and I am not aware of any that have happened where I work. But still, we read those stories avidly. Maybe we do it out of curiosity or as self-imposed cautionary tales. It may even be *schadenfreude*, that guilty pleasure of enjoying someone else's misery or its humble opposite: a dose of "there, but for the grace of God, go I." Whatever it is, the accusations and verdicts meted out make for riveting reading. There is the one we still chuckle over, about the Director of Nursing whose nursing diploma and university degrees were discovered to be fraudulent. It seems that armed with fake academic transcripts, and forged references, she managed to convince a hospital that she held an Education degree, plus a Doctorate in Nursing Science. It turned out, she had only a *lapsed* RN certificate. But, "way to go," we said, strictly in jest. You had to hand it to her – it takes some ingenuity to pull that off!

However, the vast majority of the incidents described are repugnant, even despicable. There are cases of nurses who had stolen money from patients and even one who had pilfered a patient's dentures! There were tales of nurses who had been verbally abusive to patients. One nurse was reported to have tied a nursing home resident to a toilet and left her there for hours. Another nurse had sexually assaulted a comatose patient. Even such isolated incidents reflected badly on nursing as a profession. At some time in our careers, most of us have encountered wrongdoing, either mild or severe, and each of us knows privately what we did or did not do with that information. We know whether or not we had the moral courage to stand up for what was right or whether we looked away.

But I think most of us feel proud that the College of Nurses is there to protect the public and that these complaints are out in the open. After all, we all know that transparency, reliability, integrity, and accountability are hallmarks of professionals, and if bad apples are exposed in the process, so be it.

I suggested to Jenna that we meet at a Tim Hortons coffee shop near her house. I arrived on time but she must have been there long before me as I found her poring over a thick black binder full of notes, documents, and affidavits. She looked like she was cramming for an exam. She started when I touched her shoulder. I was shocked at her appearance. She had always been slender, but now she was gaunt and looked pale and unwell. She seemed fragile and was bent forward like she had a cramp.

"I'm terrified to come back to work," she said as I brought her a cup of herbal tea and a coffee for me. "What are people saying?"

"They don't know what happened, only that you've been off work."

Jenna didn't waste a moment. She needed to share this. "When they first called me from the College of Nurses, I thought maybe I had been chosen for an award, or something," she said, slightly embarrassed. "I had no idea it was a complaint against me." She shook her head at her naïveté. "There was a friendly message on my answering machine to please call them at my earliest convenience. When I finally got back to them, they told me a family had lodged a complaint against me. By then, they had seized the chart and all I had was a faint memory of the events." I reached out to touch her hand. I wanted to offer support, but I reminded myself of the promise I made not to be swayed by emotion, to listen to all the facts as objectively as possible, and come to my own conclusions.

"Now, about the complaint itself," I said, trying to help her stay on track.

"I didn't have access to the chart but by then I had started to recall the case. It was a sixty-six-year-old woman. She was a fresh post-op repair of a perforated bowel due to an underlying malignancy. She had hypertension, diabetes, and coronary artery disease, too. Surely the family knew it was high risk surgery? She lost almost two litres of blood in the OR. Anyway, she arrested and we did a full code for more than an hour, but it was unsuccessful. She died that night on my shift but it wasn't because of anything I did or didn't do."

"Did the family say it was?"

"Not exactly . . . but they said I hadn't resuscitated her properly and that I hadn't reacted when the alarms went off. They said I had turned them off. I did turn them off, but they don't understand why. I was dealing with the problem. They also said I didn't

call the doctor soon enough and . . . they said something else."
Here Jenna fell silent, not yet ready to tell me the other thing.

We sat there for a few minutes until I prodded again. "What happened next?"

"I contacted a lawyer, even though I had to pay for it myself."

"Why? Didn't the union provide legal aid? That's what we pay our dues for, isn't it?"

"Yes, but I was afraid it wouldn't be enough and I didn't know what was involved. So far, the lawyers' fees have cost me thousands of dollars."

I looked at Jenna. I would have her as my nurse any day. But perhaps she'd been distracted by her infertility problems and not as careful or as focused? "We miss you at work," I said. "How are you managing?"

"It hasn't been easy. Technically, I can still work. I haven't been suspended because it's not a criminal trial, only an investigation of a complaint, but I haven't been feeling well. One good thing has happened during this time. I am six weeks pregnant," she said glumly. "I know I should be happy, but I'm just so stressed over this other thing that I can't even think about it. Besides, I've gotten pregnant before, but never made it past the fourth month." She sipped her tea and then looked away. "I feel very alone with all of this. I appreciate your meeting with me, Tilda. Others have called, but I just can't face them." She started to sob, but then sat up straight and blew her nose. "Okay, I'll tell you everything."

I nodded. "Yes, go on."

"When I came on to my shift that night, the patient had just arrived from the OR and I knew right away I was dealing with a very unstable patient. I asked the resident to insert a new arterial line because the one put in in the OR had a dampened waveform." She drew a diagram of the poor waveform on a paper napkin with her fingernail. "I took the patient's pressure by cuff and it was around ninety systolic, the diastolic undetectable. She was in normal sinus rhythm with a rate of about sixty-five, with no irregular beats. None." She shook her head for emphasis and took a deep gulp of air as if needing more oxygen to carry on up this mountain. "The doctor was trying to get the line in and the family kept calling from the waiting room, wanting to come in but I had a lot of work to get done first."

How well I knew this situation. Many nurses want to wipe up all the spills and messes before letting families into the room. Maybe it is because I know personally how important it is for families to be there, that I always let them in right away, especially when the patient is so critically ill. But Jenna kept them waiting and I could imagine how that might turn out to be a problem.

"Maybe you should have let them in. So what if they see the mess?" I interrupted.

"But doesn't that just add to their stress? It adds to mine because then they start freaking out and asking questions and I can't concentrate on what I'm doing for the patient."

"I know, but that's how some families grasp what's really going on."

"But doesn't there have to be *trust*?"

"I agree," I nodded. But there are some things that need to be seen to be believed, and the controlled chaos of resuscitating a patient as sick as Jenna's patient was, is hard to imagine if you've never witnessed it.

"Well, anyway, I thought I would get that arterial line secured, draw up some emergency drugs, just in case, and tidy up the room before letting them in. Meanwhile, the patient was very restless and I couldn't leave her side for a moment. She was agitated, tearing at her lines. Her abdomen was taut and distended. She was pale and clammy. I needed to draw blood work such as hemoglobin and hematocrit, since she'd lost so much blood in the OR. Her temp was high at 38.8 C and I had a peek at her X-ray and could see she was developing pneumonia, so I wanted to draw sputum and blood cultures. She was on maximum ventilator support, with one hundred per cent oxygen. I was also getting worried because she wasn't putting out much urine."

"She might have been going into pre-renal failure due to her low kidney perfusion and compromised cardiac output," I said, thinking out loud.

"That's exactly what I was thinking."

"Okay, so . . ."

"Meanwhile, the family kept calling, wanting to come in, but the patient was still thrashing around. The doctor ordered sedation, but I gave only a small dose because I was afraid it would drop her blood pressure even more. She was terribly agitated, and I tried my best to calm her down by talking to her constantly, even though she was still under the effects of the anaesthetic. I explained that if she pulled out any of her lines, she would be in grave danger. I told her that those things were helping to save her life. She kept grabbing at her tube. I asked the doctor if I could restrain her arms and he nodded okay. Then, he had to run off because he was called away to another patient. He never wrote that order and that turned out to be a problem later. Make sure you get a doctor's order for restraints, Tilda. Take it from me."

I nodded, thinking that I probably would have restrained her, too. There were many situations when restraints on the arms, and sometimes legs, too, as extreme as it sounds, did help patients through a temporary time. Sometimes, even mild-mannered people become combative when they are critically ill. I have cared for agitated patients who pulled out their arterial lines and hemorrhaged, and others who pulled out their breathing tubes and injured their airways. (I will never forget one patient in particular. She punched me in the chest and in the shoulder, and I was getting upset. Even the physiotherapist refused to treat her until she stopped being violent, but nurses can never deny someone nursing care. I had to find a way to protect myself. Reasoning with her wasn't having any effect and the sedatives were only working minimally. As a last resort, I felt I had no choice but to put soft restraints around her wrists, but that made her even more agitated. I was trying to figure out what to do when her daughter happened to call.

"My mother was a political prisoner in Argentina," she explained. "I think that's why she's so upset at being confined. If you restrain her it will only make her more frightened."

I nearly tripped over myself in my haste to remove those restraints, but by then, the patient had thoroughly exhausted herself, the sedation had kicked in, and we were both worn out.)

Jenna was ready to continue. "I was just about to call the family when they showed up at the door and barged right in. At that moment, the cardiac alarm went off and I turned and saw that the heart rate had dropped to forty-four. I ran to give her an injection of Atropine to bring the heart rate back up and while I was doing that I silenced the monitor, another thing the family later objected to. They didn't realize the problem was her low heart rate and I was treating it. Then they asked, 'Why is she tied down?' but I couldn't explain at that moment because I was busy dealing with the low heart rate. In their letter of complaint, the family claims they asked for the restraints to be removed, but I don't recall that. When families say no restraints, I always ask them to stay with the patient because I can't be there every moment to ensure the patient doesn't harm herself." Jenna looked away and tried to compose herself. This must have been what she was reluctant to mention earlier. The use of restraints is a very contentious issue.

I nodded. "It sounds like you were justified in restraining her, but let's face it, haven't you ever known a nurse who used restraints because it was easier than talking someone down or waiting for sedation to work? But anyway, go on."

"Yes, of course." She paused to find her train of thought. "But I swear to you, Tilda, I would rather face this trial than have a patient that sick yank out her airway or lines. Can you imagine if she had pulled out her endotracheal tube? We would have had to re-intubate her or even do an emergency tracheostomy that would have been even more traumatic. Can you imagine if she had pulled out her central line, how she would have bled and I would have had no intravenous access? She would have arrested without lines in place!"

We looked away from one another. This patient had died. However, had the team been unable to make every attempt to save her it would have been a worse failure. To us, restraints were the lesser of two evils, but the family clearly didn't see it that way.

"Oh, dear, who knows what is right?" Jenna said. "Here's the worst part. Just as they were getting ready to leave for the night, and I was saying to them, as I always do, that I would call if there were any changes in the patient's condition overnight, the alarm sounded and she blocked right down and went into cardiac arrest. I shooed the family out of the room and immediately started chest compressions. Casey called on the intercom for the doctor and the crash cart. He arrived about one minute later, but the family must have assumed I was doing nothing in the meantime. There was no chance to explain anything, but I could hear them outside the door getting hysterical. By then the room was packed and we were all working on her. We pulled her up and got a hard board underneath her so that the compressions would be effective. Man, they were so effective, I could hear the ribs cracking. I hate that sound, don't you?"

We both winced simultaneously at the thought. To me, what was even worse than hearing that sound was knowing that your efforts have only a slim chance of actually saving the patient.

"It was a full code. It went on for more than an hour. Each time we stopped CPR, we lost her."

Jenna stopped to take another sip of tea, even though it must have gone cold. She looked so despondent that I wasn't sure it was helping her to go over these details, but it was definitely helping me. I could picture the entire scene – the old woman intubated, her arms tied down, the stains on the bed, people pushing in syringes of drugs, and the family clamouring outside the door, angry, confused, and terrified.

"The code went on and on," Jenna had to finish the story. "I pushed epinephrine and vasopressin and we shocked her again and again. We hooked her up to an external pacemaker to buy some time. All the lines were wide open and we were pouring in drugs and fluid and all the while continuing chest compressions and ventilator breaths, switching with one another every ten minutes, so we could keep up our strength. We soon saw the direction it was going. The surgeon arrived, ready to take her back to the operating room, but by then, it was way beyond that. Her pupils were fixed and dilated. She had no heart rhythm whatsoever. When we told the family, the daughter fainted and had to be taken down to emerge."

We sat quietly together, thinking all of this over.

"Unfortunately, all of this took place right at the start of my shift." Jenna spread out her hands across all of the notes. "We hadn't had time to build up trust. I feel disappointed that our attempts to save her life aren't appreciated, but the patient was high risk to begin with. Surely they were told of the possible complications beforehand?"

She showed me the letter the family had written the College of Nurses. "What was the nurse's motive in silencing the alarm?" they'd asked. "What was she trying to hide by pushing us out of the door with no explanation of what was taking place?" they wanted to know. "The nurse gave our mother a needle, then the monitor went flat and she told us to get out. Next thing we knew the doctor came to tell us our mother was dead. Why didn't the nurse call him sooner?"

Jenna explained, "I got up on the witness stand and explained everything as best I could. Our manager attested to the fact that I was a safe nurse with a good record. The family were furious. I tried to tell them how sorry I was for their loss, but they turned away when I spoke."

"What was the outcome of the hearing?"

"It's still before the committee. They will announce their decision in a few weeks."

As we said goodbye, I hugged her and wished her good luck. We both knew, but didn't say, that if it did not go in her favour, Jenna could lose her nursing licence. I wished her well with the pregnancy and her health, because much more was at stake here than her career.

A month later, I called to see how she was doing and if she'd heard anything.

"The matter has been settled," Jenna said wearily. "At least for now."

"What do you mean?"

"The committee's decision was to take no action. They said I had not breached professional nursing standards and that I had responded in a timely and correct fashion to the emergency, but the family is appealing the ruling so the final verdict is still pending."

How conversant she had had to become in this forbidding language, relaying it without emotion, sounding neither encouraged nor vindicated, neither bitter nor disheartened, either.

"How are you feeling, Jenna?" I asked cautiously.

"I'm having problems with the pregnancy, bleeding and cramps," she said dully. "I'll be off for a while on bed rest to try to prevent a miscarriage like last time."

"You must be relieved that this trial nightmare is over."

"Yes, I am," she said quietly, unconvincingly.

I thought about all that Jenna had done and not done. In my opinion, she acted professionally and competently that night, but what she had neglected to do was let the family in immediately. Perhaps if they had seen for themselves, they would have realized that everything possible was being done to save their mother. Jenna's desire to protect the family from seeing a messy, frightening resuscitation worked against her, even though her intention was good. In the end, it was a sad story of a grief-stricken family trying to make sense of their loss and an aggrieved nurse caught in the middle. There were no winners.

Perhaps for some, the act of blaming others imparts a sense of relief. It may be that such a fight is a way for some people to honour the memory of a loved one, or is a part of their own healing process. For some people I even suspect it may be an attempt to avenge the bitter loss. But do explanations actually offer consolation? Does blame ever make anything better? I have experienced many losses, but never one that I attributed to someone else's fault, so perhaps I don't understand. I do believe that it is only by moving from anger and retribution to understanding and forgiveness that there is any hope of improving safety and building trusting relationships.

FINALLY, TIKKI RETURNED from her vacation. We arranged to meet on a day that we both had off work, away from the ICU but at the hospital Starbucks kiosk, rather than at the usual Tim Hortons (or "Timmie Ho's," as some call it) because they had more comfortable chairs. Most nurses drank Tim Hortons on the run and if they preferred the darker roasts at Starbucks, it was always "to go." In between cases, doctors may be able to make time to meet for coffee and others do so in between meetings, but for nurses, our time is not our own and we can't run off from our patients, sit and linger over café lattes at these blond wood tables, listening to piped-in jazz in the middle of the afternoon. Our work rarely allowed time for reflective pauses or discussions unless we arranged for it after hours, on our own time. As I waited for Tikki, I looked around. Sitting at the other tables were managers and administrators, wearing stylish suits and jackets of sophisticated hues. I overheard one telling the others that she had observed a nurse standing outside a patient's door checking off a list of tasks. "Tick, tick, tick," she said contemptuously. "Is that all nurses do nowadays?"

Tikki arrived and apologized for being late. She pulled her earphones out and sat down. "Wassup?" She seemed puzzled.

"Tikki," I started. "You've been in the ICU five months. How do you like it?"

"It's awesome. I love it. You've been a big help, Tilda. I really appreciate it."

"How do you think you're doing?" I saw she had no idea that there was a problem. I took a deep breath. "Tikki, I have serious concerns about your work." She looked shocked at the suggestion that her practice was other than impeccable. I spread out my notes on the table so we could look at them together. Her bad-girl tattoos and cocky manner now seemed like so much bravado. She looked like a lost little girl. I steeled myself to present my long list of complaints. When I came to the end, Tikki was no longer surprised or bewildered. She was enraged. She stood up.

"Fuck you, Tilda! You're trying to ruin my career! I've only worked in the ICU such a short time and you haven't stopped picking on me. Give me a break! These are such little things you're finding fault with. This is harassment! I'm going to take it to the union and file a grievance against you." She spat out the words at me. I sat there in silence and accepted the venom. It was such a small price to pay for the satisfaction of doing the right thing.

13

CHESS MOVES

"Remember the days when we used to work in teams?" Noreen asked. We were sitting in the staff lounge and had a few more minutes before we had to get back to our patients. I looked at her over the top of my newspaper. "Do I remember? How could I ever forget? Those women are my sisters."

Christmas had been the last time I'd seen them. Now it was February and my birthday was coming up, so I knew we'd be getting together soon.

"You were on Laura's Line, weren't you?" Noreen asked. "Did Laura become a doctor?"

"No, that didn't pan out, but she acts like one and still bosses doctors around."

"Tracy was part of your team, too, wasn't she, but what about the others?"

"Frances works with Laura in an out-patient clinic, assisting with angiograms and biopsies. Nicky moved to the States with her husband. She's still a scratch golfer and now has three kids and works part-time in a cardiovascular ICU."

"What about Justine? Now, there was a real go-to kind of gal! I always thought she would become a lawyer or go into politics. What a great sense of humour she had. Once, I got on an elevator with her and she called out, 'Let me off at the liposuction suite!' Everyone was in stitches!"

"Justine also has three kids. She's a hockey mom, plays baseball on a women's team, and has her own business. She's doing great and looks fantastic."

ON THE SATURDAY closest to my birthday, we met for afternoon tea at a funky, bohemian place on Queen Street called the Red Tea Box.

"Who chose *this* joint?" Justine asked, rolling her eyes.

"Tilda, of course," Laura gestured at me. "It's artsy-fartsy."

"Hey Tilda, are you and Tracy still torturing people in the ICU?" Justine asked. "D'you guys remember that patient's son who called Tilda the Angel of Death? Say, isn't it time to move on from the ICU? Haven't you had enough?"

"Not yet. I still haven't figured it all out," I said.

"If that's the case, then you'll never leave." Justine shook her head in amazement. "I can't believe you two still work there. Do the families still call the shots and demand everything be done before their loved one croaks? If those patients could talk, they'd beg for a visit from Dr. Kevorkian!"

"Do you guys remember that patient's wife with the weird hair that was all teased and matted?" I asked. "The one that Justine threatened, 'I'm going to hold you upside down and use you for a mop!' and instead of being insulted, she howled with laughter."

We remembered that – and much more. I looked around the table at them and silently hoped there would be mentors like them for new nurses coming along. I told them about Tikki, how angry she was and how she was threatening to make trouble for me with the union.

Laura didn't need a moment to think it over. "Get rid of her. Make sure she doesn't come anywhere near patients. You have a responsibility to see she gets the boot."

"She said I wasn't giving her a chance and that I was trying to ruin her career."

"Suck it up, princess. Get over it. The stakes are too high in the ICU to mess around."

"I have to agree," said Tracy quietly. "She's a scary nurse."

Only Frances felt differently. "Don't give up on her, Tilda," she advised. "Not just yet. Maybe she just needs more time buddied with you." I suddenly remembered how hard Frances had worked with me and how patient she had been with me in my early ICU days. It was unthinkable to Frances to give up on someone. "Tell her you're prepared to keep working with her and point out where she needs to improve. Oh, geez, I'm having a hot flash." Frances pulled out a fan and flapped it madly at her face.

We *were* getting older, weren't we?

"It used to be all you had to say was 'panties' to make Frances blush," chortled Justine. "Hey, Frances, have you been following the case of the Recipe Robber? There's this thief who goes around making demands for cash on the back of recipe cards. 'Gimme $1,000,000' on one side and 'Mom's Chocolate Cake' on the other!"

Frances had a predilection for collecting recipes, following weird crimes in the news, and reading the obituary column in the newspaper too, word for word.

"Mmm . . . chocolate reminds me of Nell's classic candy diagnosis," Laura said with glee.

(I don't think we'd ever gotten together and not exchanged tales of our colleague super-nurse Nell Mason, whose legend lives on, long after her untimely death.)

"That was one of my faves," I chuckled, but Tracy didn't remember it so Justine filled her in.

"That was when Nell was running an Emergency depart-ment single-handedly and a woman came in with an unusual gynecological problem. Nell figured out she'd stuck a Mars Bar up there!"

"The tip-off must have been the nougat and caramel dripping down her legs," said Laura dryly, with a snort of contempt for Nell's outrageous confabulations, her brilliance as a nurse notwith-standing.

Justine remembered another tall tale. "How about when Nell
was an outpost nurse on a native reserve, delivering babies and
performing appendectomies – according to her – and this old Cree
woman came in with a foul stench? Nell examined her and found
a festering crow inside of her. She said she had to remove feathers
and little bones."

"What about her claim that she never went to the bathroom
at the hospital in all her years working there? I suppose she
adopted the water-retention ability of her pet camel," Laura said,
"the one she used to ride to school, dontcha remember? Imagine,
riding a camel in Thunder Bay! Did she really think we believed
those stories? Hey, did she ever tell you about her practice
of scatomancy?"

"What the hell is that?" asked Justine.

"She claimed she could tell people's fortunes by examining their
feces."

"Eeewww!" we all exclaimed, laughing helplessly.

"Well, I always said old Nell was full of shit," scoffed Laura,
but then looked a bit remorseful for making fun of Nell once again.
I think we all regretted that we hadn't recognized that Nell was
seriously ill. In the end she died at home alone, after a long and
private battle with alcoholism.

"None of us ever really knew the late, great Nell Mason," I said.

"Yes," said Justine sincerely. "Nell was Über-Nurse."

"Let's have cake," said Frances. "It's Tilda's birthday."

THE NEXT DAY AT WORK, Tikki was back and I found a moment
to speak with her privately. "Listen, Tikki, if you are willing,
we can continue to work together and if we review some
of the . . ."

She shook her head. "At first I was upset with you, Tilda. I don't
usually let anyone push me around like that and I really took it
hard but now I feel, *whatever*." She gave a wave of indifference.
"I've decided to go back to school for my Master's in Nursing, so
I can teach or do research."

I was blown away. Did I look as astonished as I felt?

"Don't worry, it's no biggie," she said with a shrug and worked her last shift without incident.

I wasn't sorry to see Tikki go but we *had* been losing a lot of nurses lately. Chandra had left and Jenna was still off work for health reasons. Monica would soon complete her Master's degree and was already looking for a position in management. Even Tracy had been thinking of moving on and trying something different, such as public health nursing, after nearly twenty years in the ICU. The loss of experienced nurses had been putting a real stress on the ICU. We were short-staffed on almost every shift and sick-time and overtime costs were cutting deeply into the budget. The ICU had been crazy-busy for more than a year and we'd been working non-stop. The moment one patient was discharged, another was right there. Nurses were complaining they were feeling like factory workers on an assembly line, trying to keep up with the pace that showed no signs of letting up.

It was easy to see why more patients needed to come to the ICU. You only had to walk through the wards to see that the floor patients were sicker than ever. In today's hospitals, patients who used to be treated on the floors are now being discharged home "sicker and quicker," nurses on the floor always say. More and more, patients who are in the hospital need closer monitoring, quicker intervention, and the attention to detail that we are able to provide in the ICU.

We had long since moved from both the original ten-bed ICU where I had started (memories of the Cave) and then a few years later, from a sixteen-bed ICU in another part of the hospital. About three years ago we moved into a bright, spacious new twenty-two-bed ICU, up on the tenth floor, with a view of the city right down to the lakeshore. In this ICU, there are large patient rooms, expansive hallways with turquoise and beige geometrical designs on the floors, and windows all around that let in not only light, but also a sense of space and grandeur, as well as glimpses of the outside world. It is a much more pleasant place than the original ICU. Back then ten beds had been sufficient, but now we are always full to overflowing with twenty-two beds. More and more patients need to come to the ICU.

Is the ICU a physical place or a way of doing things? I got to thinking about this question after what happened to a patient named Carole Oxton. She was not my patient but was Xavier's in the room next door to mine. However, as the day went on and I saw what was unfolding, I had no choice but to get involved. Noreen, Casey, and Monica were on that day, too, and Roberta was in charge. I had worked with Xavier a few times and I had no concerns about him. He was a new nurse, but very competent and caring and what I liked about him was that he asked a lot of questions and that's always a good sign. He was assigned to care for Carole Oxton because she was a stable patient. In fact, she was deemed so stable she was to be transferred out of the ICU early that afternoon. She was a fifty-four-year-old woman with a long history of alcohol and drug abuse who had fallen down a flight of stairs at home and broken her arm. She had dark circles around her eyes (even textbooks labelled them "raccoon eyes") and multiple purple bruises all over her body. Her electrolytes – the potassium, sodium, calcium, magnesium, and phosphate levels in her blood – were abnormal due to liver and kidney failure. They needed to be closely monitored and swiftly treated, in order to avoid serious complications. I saw that Xavier was very capably topping up the low phosphate and preparing to give a calcium supplement, so I returned to my patient in the room next door.

Mr. Drummond was a sixty-year-old man, three days post lung-transplant, weaning slowly off the ventilator, getting used to his new lungs and battling re-perfusion syndrome.[*] On rounds that morning, we tweaked his medications on the advice of the pharmacist. On the respiratory therapist's recommendations, we adjusted the ventilator so as to allow him to gradually do more of the "work of breathing," by himself. He was making progress, but still had a long way to go.

The team pushed the portable computer along to the next room, Mrs. Oxton's.

"This lady is doing well," said the resident. "She's ready to be transferred to the floor." Since no one had anything to add, they

---

[*] This syndrome is a common, but complicated, risk post lung-transplant.

moved on to the next patient. Yet, after a mere glance at Mrs. Oxton, I felt uneasy and clearly, Xavier did too. "I don't think she's ready to be transferred out," he said.

"She's been off the ventilator for forty-eight hours," the resident called back over his shoulder. "Her blood gases are good. She's a rose. She could have gone out yesterday."

"It's true," said Xavier, thinking out loud to me. "She's on nasal prongs with just a few litres of oxygen, but the problem is, she's not very alert. I don't have a good feeling about her."

"How's her blood pressure?" I asked, trying to figure out what it was that disturbed me, too.

"Normal," Xavier said, looking unhappy. "What do you think, Tilda?"

"Let's go in and examine her together," I suggested.

Xavier's patient opened her eyes when she saw us. She made raspy gurgles of secretions at the back of her throat. I handed her a tissue. "Try to cough that out."

"I've paid my bills," she mumbled. She tried to cough, but only managed a feeble splutter. Even without listening with my stethoscope, I could hear her chest was noisy.

"Mrs. Oxton!" I shook her shoulder a little. "Would you like to get out of bed?" She didn't answer or even appear to have heard me. I looked at Xavier.

"I already tried to sit her up at the side of the bed and dangle her legs," he explained, "but she was too weak to stand."

"Let's hoist her up," I said, "it'll make it easier for her to breathe." Xavier went on the other side of the bed and we lifted her as she lay there helplessly.

"If we had extra staff, we could keep her longer," Roberta said when I went to the nurses' station to talk to her about it, "but as it is I am short two nurses and three short for the night shift."

"We always have to move everyone along so fast," I grumbled.

"I know how you feel, but we're getting two transplants and someone just called in sick." Roberta stared into the staffing book as if more nurses would suddenly materialize in there. "Hey, it's still early. We'll keep her a few more hours and reassess the situation in the afternoon."

I'm convinced the best preparation for this role would be to study the moves of the grand chess masters, Kasparov, Fischer, and Spassky and so on. The nurse in charge has to control the board (the ICU) and plan moves (transfers, discharges, room swaps, etc.) in advance. You have to stay a few steps ahead and have a strategy for a possible arrest on the floor, or a surprise admission from the Emergency department. You have to be ready to move some "pieces" out quickly and hold others back and protect them. The King is your sickest patient, but you also have to protect your Queen – your last ICU bed. Roberta was a supreme chess master, and in her hands, the ICU could cope with any "attack."

About an hour or so later, I wandered back to the nurses' station to get a sense of how the game was playing out. Roberta looked stressed. "I see you're 'Takin' Care of Business,'" I sang, trying to play our old game, but she wasn't in the mood. I could see by her expression that it was time for push to come to shove, quite literally.

Roberta looked at me. "Mrs. Oxton has to go, Tilda. There's a patient on the floor who is deteriorating fast and needs to come to the ICU. I want you to help Xavier get her ready to be transferred out." She returned to the lists of nurses and patients and tried to massage the numbers to stretch the supply of staff to cover the demand of patients, all the while doing her utmost to ensure everyone would be safe. "Let's see," I heard her talking to herself, "if we transfer the patient in 1011 out, then Casey can take the liver transplant when he comes out of the OR and when Xavier's patient goes out, we'll admit the floor patient . . ."

"Why did you agree to stay open to admissions if you're so short of nurses?" asked Dr. Sandor, as he passed by the nurses' station. He helped himself to a squirt of antibacterial lotion.

"How could I say no?" Roberta asked in dismay.

"But it's a staffing issue. That's your call. Take a stand."
Check.

"And I suppose you'll back me up when the newspaper headline tomorrow reads, 'ICU Closes Doors due to Shortage of Nurses'?"

She glared at him and he grinned back. "That's what I thought," she said.

Checkmate.

I COULD SEE THE PRESSURE Roberta was under, but still I stalled, trying to buy more time for Mrs. Oxton in the ICU. Xavier and I fussed around her and turned the radio on to stimulate her. We tried again to get her out of bed, but she became combative. We wondered if she might be starting to go through the DT's,[*] the syndrome of agitated withdrawal from alcohol. I sat down to read her chart. She had been a widow for many years and had a teenaged son who was in jail. Three days ago a neighbour found her lying unconscious on the floor of her basement apartment. Empty liquor bottles were strewn about.

"I heard you are planning to transfer Carole out," said a thin, anxious woman who came up from behind me. She frowned and then introduced herself as Margaret, Mrs. Oxton's sister.

"She is ready to be transferred out," I said uneasily.

"Someone else needs the bed, is that it?" she asked.

I squirmed, but by my silence, she knew the answer. Xavier stood by, listening in.

"The nursing care is better here in the ICU. I know it and you do, too."

"She will be well taken care of by the nurses on the floor," I said. *Of course she would, she and another six equally needy patients that some nurse would be running back and forth between.* I recalled a patient I transferred out of the ICU a few weeks ago. He was a renal patient on dialysis three times a week who was recovering from septic shock. He was confused and disoriented and on top of all of that, he spoke only Italian so I could not communicate with him properly. On the floor, I gave a report to a nurse who was listening but in a very distracted way. "The other thing," I added at the end, loath to add to her burden, "you'll need to get hold of

---

[*] Delirium tremens.

an interpreter so you can explain his meds. Could you page one?"
I asked the ward clerk who was listening in.

"This isn't the UN," she grumbled, then tried to be helpful.
"How about, 'Hey *Paisano!*'"

"How many other patients do you have?" I asked the nurse.

"Along with this one? Seven. No, wait a sec," she reviewed her
notes. "Six. One just died." She crossed a name off her list.

"Are all of them this sick?"

She nodded. I noticed she was panting and looked as if she was
ready to take off on a sprint.

"Why are you so short of breath?" She worried me.

"From running. A patient just yanked out his chest tube and
then the patient in the other bed took out a knife and cut his own
chest tubes off."

"Were they psychotic?"

"No, just competing with one another." I couldn't tell if she was
joking or not.

"You look stressed," I said. All of a sudden, she got up and ran
into a patient's room. My patient – the one she'd just inherited
from me – was climbing out of bed. How did she even know?
Together, we lugged his heavy, swollen legs back into bed, and I
put the side rails back up.

Good night, nurse! I thought, walking away from her, feeling
guilty leaving her with such a mess. *Good luck!* I am ashamed to
admit how fast I booted it out of there and raced back to the ICU.
It was my home and while there was chaos there too, at times, we
had the ways and means to tame it.

Now I understood what was the biggest dilemma for nurses.
We can no longer solely focus on doing good for patients. We are
doing everything in our power to ensure we don't cause them harm.

"The nurses on the floor won't have time for her," Margaret,
the sister, said.

"Yes, they will," I lied.

"She is falling off a cliff," she said. "Do something!"

Xavier removed Carole's arterial line, and I gathered up her personal belongings. There wasn't much, only a dirty pair of jeans,

old running shoes, a T-shirt, and a grimy jacket. I placed them in a plastic bag and tried to give it to her sister to take home, but she wouldn't touch it.

"I've spoken to my son who is a doctor, and he insists Carole stay in the ICU. This is a disgrace."

"I understand how you feel." I felt the same way.

"We have a terrible health-care system."

Just then, a teenaged boy bolted into the room. "I'm the son," he said, slamming his jacket onto a coat hook so violently it ripped right off the wall.

Margaret whispered, "I didn't know whether to tell him to come. He's out on probation."

"Is she even with it?" the son said, staring at his dishevelled mother, who was grinning and gurgling, sprawled in the bed, not appearing to recognize him one bit. "She's a drunk," he said in disgust, "plus she's a junkie, so it's no use trying to save her because she'll just be back again in a few days."

"Don't you think you should take her for a CT scan?" Margaret inquired politely. "When my husband got sick, they took him for a CT and it helped him get better."

Out in the hall, Noreen asked me, "Why do you let your patient's sister boss you around?" Everyone was watching this drama play out.

"She has to go," Roberta came over to tell me. She had paged housekeeping to clean the room that hadn't even been vacated yet. Roberta knew the bigger picture and this patient and her sister were the smaller picture. Just one little patient caught in the big scheme of a huge and mighty hospital.

"Carole!" Xavier and I shouted at her, trying to make her more alert. If she was more alert, she might be able to protect her airway from aspiration. "Carole, wake up. Open your eyes."

"The fishing rod is too tight," Carole muttered, pulling at her central line, the IV in the jugular vein in her neck. "I can't reel it in."

The housekeeper arrived and started cleaning the floor around her bed, then stopped and leaned on her mop. "This patient is going to the floor? She don't look too good."

"See, even *she* can see it," exclaimed Margaret. "Have the courage to stand up for her! Where's a doctor? Get a doctor!"

I would gladly call the doctor if she wanted, but it was a nursing matter, pure and simple. Pure, perhaps, but not so simple.

"Who changed the time for transportation?" I heard Roberta ask. Sneakily, behind her back, I had rebooked the porter in order to buy more time. Roberta was getting frustrated with me, as were other nurses. Word was getting around the unit that I was not supporting our charge nurse, that I was getting too emotional and not taking a firm enough hand with a demanding family member. Roberta came over and spoke to me sternly. "Tilda, we can't keep Xavier's patient here any longer."

Margaret, in turn, confronted Roberta. "You know very well she should stay, but you're feeling pressure to move her along and bring someone else in. If she dies, it will be on your conscience. Please do the right thing and keep her here."

"I can't," Roberta said, throwing her hands up in the air.

Margaret crossed her arms across her chest and looked away, fuming.

"I suggest if you are concerned about your sister that you stay with her on the floor," Roberta advised. "That's what I would do if someone I loved was in the hospital. This is what we are dealing with right now in our health-care system. Choices have to be made."

Roberta and I stepped out into the hallway to discuss the matter further. "Look, Tilda, the nurses downstairs will be able to handle this patient. I know she has a lot of needs, but what can we do?"

The resident came over. "I've written the transfer orders. She's good to go."

Well, what could we do in the meantime, but go for our lunch breaks? There had been a meeting of the managers that day, and there were sandwiches and éclairs. I had to chuckle at Casey, who was serving the Caesar salad, using tongue depressors as tongs.

"I can't stand the waste of money," Monica said and looked at the fancy leftovers with disgust while we munched away. "Everyone knows our health-care system is in trouble."

"Oh, come on, Monica. There are lots worse excesses. A few platters of food is a drop in the bucket," I snapped. She was ruining my appetite with her griping, and that on top of my *real* problem. "I've got bigger issues on my mind."

"Why are you being so difficult, Tilda?" she asked. "You know there's another patient out there who is in worse shape."

"I realize that!" I could hear a hysterical edge to my voice. "But don't we also have a responsibility to the patient already in our care?"

"But that other patient deserves a chance at what the ICU has to offer, too," Monica said. "It's not like we're sending her home. Don't underestimate the nurses on the floor."

"You know as well as I do that a patient like this can easily fall between the cracks."

"Look, if the family is giving you a problem, call security."

And smash this tiny ant with a sledgehammer? Was that the solution? How easy it was for them all to weigh in on the matter. Why was it never so easy for me?

"Xavier," I said briskly when I came back, "I'm going to help you transfer this patient."

He looked surprised at my change of heart.

"What!" shouted Margaret, who was sitting beside the bed.

"Your sister cannot stay in the ICU."

"You know what the right thing to do is, you are just not willing to do it." Her eyes bored into me. "Look at her! She's so frail. Imagine it was *your* sister. Please, keep her here," Margaret pleaded.

"Unfortunately, we can't," I said crisply as I disconnected the patient from the cardiac monitor.

"I suppose you have someone sicker who you want to bring in her place," Margaret sniffed.

I didn't dare tell her she was right, but Roberta came over and she dared. "Yes, that's exactly what is happening. Someone is in worse shape than your sister."

Check.

The porter arrived. Xavier released the brake on the bed. As we wheeled the bed out of the ICU, I fought back tears of rage at what we were forced to do.

Checkmate.

I HONESTLY CAN'T SAY I was shocked when I came back to work the next morning and heard that Carole Oxton had a respiratory arrest during the night and had to be brought back to the ICU, unconscious and re-intubated. I'm not even certain the wrong decision was made to transfer her out, given that our resources are not unlimited. We can't always keep patients in the ICU because of the *possibility* that something could go wrong. But I did wish that it were possible for nurses all over the hospital to be in the position to give the kind of care that we give to our patients. The hospital is full of seriously ill people and don't they all deserve *intensive care*? After all, what was most "intensive" and "caring" about the ICU was the nurses. It wasn't merely a place with machines and equipment; it was a way of doing things. And since it wasn't feasible to bring every patient to the ICU, perhaps there was some way that we could bring the ICU to patients?

14

INHOSPITABLE HOSPITALS

S uddenly, my life became more complicated. After standing by helplessly and watching what happened to Carole Oxton, I felt terribly disheartened. We hadn't been able to keep her safe. We couldn't do the right thing for her. All around me, I began to see more and more things I could no longer ignore. Nurses on the floor were overloaded and distressed. There was no one they could turn to for support or to ask questions. Nurses were leaving nursing, and I was beginning to understand why. Jessica, a friend of mine, left nursing. She became a nurse when she was in her mid-thirties, after a successful career as a musician in the symphony. But after less than a year in the workplace, she decided to leave the profession. She looked miserable and defeated as she told me about it.

"I felt I had no choice but to walk away. Can you understand, Tilda?" She felt she had to explain it to me, but I knew very well that hospitals could be very *inhospitable* places, not only for patients, but also for conscientious nurses like Jessica. "Patients were always dissatisfied with me because I wasn't giving enough care to them, but I was always off somewhere else, giving not enough care to another patient."

"I guess you never had a chance to get to know your patients," I murmured.

"Know them? I was lucky if I knew their names. All I knew was their room numbers."

Why had I never walked away? I had been tempted long ago, when I worked on the floor and always felt so powerless and invisible. I had chalked it up to my personal problems at the time, but what if I went back to the floor now? I'm still not sure I could handle the conditions there. More than ever, I appreciated working in the ICU. We could set goals, plan ahead, intervene early, and not always be scrambling to react to crises. As an ICU nurse you felt respected, that your voice was heard and that your contribution counted. I was beginning to realize that many nurses out there didn't feel that way.

These impossible situations made me worry about my profession, but even more, about patients who don't have enough nursing care. I didn't know what to do, but I knew I couldn't look away any more. (Of course it wasn't all up to me to rescue the patients, save the hospital, and fix the problems in the health-care system, but at times, I felt like it was!)

I have never had a problem or a worry, either big or small, that couldn't be made better by meeting with a girlfriend and talking about it over coffee. If only world leaders could do the same, I'm certain wars could be averted. I arranged to meet Monica at a café near her gym just before her spinning class. I knew she was finishing up her Master's degree and I wanted to hear how that was going, but first, she was bursting to tell me about her thrilling love life that involved yet another married doctor.

"But what happened with you and Nick?" I asked. I thought he was steady at the time, but it was hard to keep track as she always had a steady and one or two on the side.

"Oh, Nick is strictly PG-13," she said. "You won't believe who I'm seeing now!"

Suddenly, I was disgusted with myself. I'd been listening to her stories for years and here I was, listening once again, to the titillating details of her latest encounter, this one in the office of a prominent surgeon, while his waiting room filled up with patients. "He said to me, 'For years, I've been dying to get my hands on you, Monica,' and so you know what I said to him? 'Well, then, do me.' We had to stop when his secretary knocked on the door."

I felt queasy. By listening, I was drawn in. I became a part of her deception.

"I'm having such fun." Monica sighed and smiled to herself. She explained how she had to be unfettered by emotional commitment so she could focus on her career goals. I looked at her pretty face and her impossibly fit body with its perfect posture from years at Catholic school where nuns had tied a broomstick to her back to make her sit up straight. She was determined to have a fabulous career and fun on her own terms, but I wondered if she really could manage to "have it all."

"How's work going?" I asked. "You haven't been in the ICU for a while."

"I've been moonlighting at another hospital," she said. "You wouldn't believe what happened the other night. They sent me to a floor and I got a fresh post-op patient who wasn't peeing. The doctor told me not to put a urinary catheter in, but after a few hours she still wasn't peeing and I needed to get a better assessment of her fluid balance. So I decided to put one in anyway and . . ."

"I hope you didn't do it, Monica, not against a doctor's order."

"It was political," she said, avoiding my question. "The doctor said she'd be more alert by morning and wouldn't need a catheter, but in the meanwhile she had zip urine output and I was worried. I was there with the patient. He was on his cell phone at home."

"Yeah, and if you had put one in and the patient had developed a urinary tract infection or blood in her urine, your licence would have been on the line."

"But he was digging his heels in and it was about power, not about what was best for the patient. I told him to get in here and see for himself. So, he came in and to be honest, he took one look at me and didn't give me any further hassles about the patient. He invited me into his on-call room and, well . . ."

"Don't tell me!" I interrupted. "You didn't!"

"He said, 'You're so hot, Monica,' and so I locked the door and we made out a bit on the couch and then I told him he was wrong about the catheter, and about a few other things, too, and he was pretty weakened at that point, and gave in to me. Anyway, the point is, I can't stand it when a nurse sees a problem, knows what to do, but her hands are tied."

She may have meant that literally. She had a penchant for kinky things and did take pride in her claim that she'd try anything once. She looked pleased with herself, as much for having fought for what she believed was best for the patient, as for making another conquest along the way.

I got up to leave. Monica looked surprised. "Why are you going so soon? We didn't even get to what you wanted to talk about." I had had enough. Monica was so completely at ease with her secret, lying life and relentless pursuit of pleasure that it brought her integrity into question – and mine, too. Who Monica was as a person tainted who she was as a nurse. I no longer respected her or valued her opinions.

I WANTED TO SEE how Chandra was doing and we arranged to meet. She had been a fabulous critical care nurse, but never regained her confidence after making that terrible medication error. Her new job was in a five-bed ICU in a small community hospital in the suburbs. She said she chose it for the convenience of being closer to home, but I think she may also have been hoping it would be a less stressful environment. She soon discovered that even there the issues were just as big and the stakes just as high.

"I have to tell you what happened on my last shift," Chandra said, launching right into the story. "A sixty-year-old man came in with pneumonia. On my shift he developed chest pain and I saw ST wave changes on the monitor that could indicate ischemia to the heart, so I gave him oxygen by nasal prongs, did a twelve-lead ECG, and called the staff doctor at home to tell him what was going on, but he just blew me off. 'He doesn't have a cardiac history,' he says. 'It's respiratory. I'll see him in the morning.' But I had an uneasy feeling and so I called him back at two and then again at two-thirty and by four, after a whole night of pressuring him, he finally came in. By then the patient was in really bad shape. He said, 'Chandra, I want to speak with you privately.' Okay, this is it, I thought. What's he going to do? He's either going to rake me over the coals or report me to the College of Nurses. He stood there, looking from side to side. He couldn't face me. 'Okay,' he said. 'Help me. What should I do?' That broke the tension a bit, and then I told him, 'Make some calls and have the patient transferred immediately to a cardiac centre.' So then, he goes out and tells the family about life support and scares them to death, but this is someone we can actually save – that part he forgot to mention. I hear them saying, 'No, Dad wouldn't want to be kept alive if he was a vegetable.' So I explained it to them. 'No, it's not like that at all. It would be a temporary measure to get him through this crisis. We only want to transfer him out so that we'll have a chance to save him.'"

"What happened?"

"I got him transferred out. He had a massive heart attack, but last I heard he's improving." She looked me in the eyes. "Why don't they listen to us?" she asked, as if I knew.

"What's the answer?" I asked, as if she knew.

ABOUT TWO YEARS AGO, people with minds much greater than mine must have been seeing the same problems I was seeing because they came up with the idea to create a mobile team of doctors and nurses that would scout out patients in trouble wherever they were in the hospital and nip problems in the bud. Nurses and doctors could page the team at any time and an ICU nurse would be the first responder on the scene. Not every patient could come to the ICU, but the ICU (at least, what it provides) could come to every patient in the hospital who needed it. It would be like a virtual ICU, an ICU without walls, they said. (They had recently created a Virtual Library at the hospital where you could access the library materials wherever you were, regardless of library hours, and without the need to physically go to a place where the materials existed in hard copy.)

A virtual ICU would be here, there, and everywhere and the nurses
would be the driving forces behind it. The nurses chosen for the
team were some of the best of the ICU and they even underwent
additional preparation and examinations on making patient
assessments, interpreting cardiac rhythms, treating electrolyte
imbalances, and instituting emergency procedures.

What a great idea, I thought, because even if I hadn't read all
the studies – which I had – I knew that nurses saved lives. Actually,
I'd realized that truth instantly, years ago, when Justine walked in
wearing a T-shirt that said, "Nurses – there to save your ass, not
kiss it."

MEANWHILE, IN THE ICU, major changes were underway. Dr.
Sandor took us all by surprise one morning with the announcement
that he wanted the nurses to take charge of morning rounds. The
nurses would present their patients' medical history and results of
diagnostic tests. He wanted the nurses to draw conclusions and not
merely rhyme off the numbers, but rather, "To do something with
those numbers and put the whole picture together." Dr. Sandor had
always been disappointed in nurses who didn't make a significant
contribution on rounds or who didn't take initiative with their
patient care. But, he had always consistently believed in us even
when we didn't believe in ourselves. Time and time again he threw
down the gauntlet of taking on bigger challenges in our practice.
He'd always been our strongest supporter, yet not everyone realized it. I'd watched him take aside a group of residents on their first
day in the ICU and tell them, "Listen to the nurses. They know
everything about the patient and you'll learn the most from them."

"It's time the nurses took on more of a leadership role," he told
us in a meeting.

"More work?" some complained bitterly.

"We're not doctors," others objected. "Is he expecting us to be
doctors as well as nurses?"

Over the years, nurses had been taking on more and more of the
tasks doctors used to perform and most saw this as an advancement

and enjoyed those added responsibilities, but clearly not all saw it that way.

I remembered a night I was working and a young woman arrested. We tried for two hours to resuscitate her. The husband and her family were in the waiting room, hoping for good news. At midnight, we called off the code – I remember because the time of death was exactly 0000 hours. The doctor looked at me. "I have to go out there and tell them, don't I?" He was inexperienced and scared. He had never broken such terrible news. Also, he didn't have a relationship with the patient or her family. On the other hand, I did. She was a high school teacher and I had often brought her two young children in from the waiting room to visit her. I had spoken many times with her husband, a dentist. "How about we go together?" I suggested. "I'll tell them, but it will mean a lot if you're there, too." He said he couldn't go. He had to write orders and there was a dialysis line to put in. What did I need him for, he asked? Couldn't I do it on my own? I recalled a conversation I'd had with him a few days ago when I'd asked him out of interest, as I always do, what he was planning to specialize in. "Nuclear cardiology," he'd said. He was adept at procedures and probably got top marks in biochemistry and physics. He would make a good scientist. (Tracy and I stifled our giggles the time he'd asked during rounds, "When's lunch?" and the staff doctor shot him a withering glance.)

As I walked out to the waiting room, I moved extra-slowly, trying to draw out the time when the family could still believe they had a wife and a mother. No, not everyone had the tact or maturity to deliver bad news, but I knew that I did, and that night, I did it the best I could.

I wanted Dr. Sandor to clarify his new plan for rounds. "What, exactly, are you asking the nurses to do? Some of them are unsure about their new responsibilities."

He looked at me in exasperation. "It's not rocket science. I want the nurses to take the lead. They will present the medical history, review the systems – cardiac, respiratory, and so forth – and highlight the problems. I want the nurses to interpret the data, spot trends, suggest approaches. They can do more than merely rattle off the numbers from the flow sheet."

Even Tracy had reservations. "What if I miss something important?" she asked, though she was one of the nurses least likely to miss anything.

"They don't pay me enough to take on even more responsibilities," one of the others said.

"I can't understand why this is so radical," Dr. Sandor said. For years, he'd been trying to get us to take ownership of our practice. Whenever it was decided that a patient was not to be resuscitated – a DNR status – and we asked Dr. Sandor to write that in the chart, he would refuse. "If the nurse knows the patient's wishes, a doctor's order is not required. The nurse knows the right thing to do."

"But we need it in writing," we insisted.

"Nonsense," he said, and showed us a copy of the policy from our own College of Nurses that clearly stated that nurses could act independently in these situations in accordance with what they knew were the patient's wishes. He was getting impatient with us and was baffled that some nurses were reluctant to jump at the opportunity he felt he was offering. Here he was endorsing our profession, much to our protest.

THE ICU OUTREACH TEAM was now in place. Nurses were roving all around the hospital, responding to problems and dealing with them on the spot. They told me what they were seeing.

"On the floors, it's mostly junior nurses. There's no one they can ask questions or look up to," George said. "One nurse told me she'd never changed a chest tube drain and she had four full ones, so I did it with her. I was with a nurse when a patient arrested and it was her first code so I showed her how to push the IV drugs."

"I think they feel that now they have someone to call, someone nonjudgmental who won't give them a hard time," Tracy told me.

"It infuriates me how doctors don't listen to nurses! We all know that can be lethal," Roberta told me, "but I see it, time and time again, especially on the floor."

"Yeah," I agreed, "but what's worse is when nurses don't speak up in the first place."

The outreach team had only been in place for a few months when a patient came in to visit. I didn't recognize him at first and asked if I could help him. When he told me he was Mr. Spruce who had undergone a lung transplant a few months ago, I gasped. Here was this man looking so healthy and vibrant. I had only known him intubated and unconscious. He wanted to thank us all, but particularly Tracy, who wasn't on that day. "Do you want to leave her a message?" I handed him a paper and a pen.

"It's a hard thing to put in a note," he said with a wry smile. "How do you thank someone for saving your life?" As he started to tell his story, people gathered around him in the hallway.

"I could feel myself going down. I now believe I was close to death. I barely had the strength for the next breath. Nurses were all hovering around me, but didn't know what to do. They were waiting for the doctor. Someone went to find one and then I was left alone. I could feel myself losing consciousness. When Tracy arrived, I immediately remembered her from the ICU. She didn't say much, but she knew exactly what she was doing. I could feel her rescuing me. She put in an IV and poured in fluid. I felt myself coming alive again. I don't know what else she did, but I know she saved my life. Please tell her when you see her."

Yeah, I'll tell her. Hey Tracy, you're not just a pretty face and a kind heart. You saved someone's life.

The outreach team, a "flying squad of experts," as one hospital official called it, was working out well. The staff doctors said the ICU nurses were like another pair of eyes and ears on the floor. One said it was like having a medical resident on the floor, taking care of everything. The floor nurses appreciated the support the ICU nurses were offering. Patients and families were already feeling and noticing the improvements. However, there was one recurring and troubling note of discontent among the nurses.

"Why should I take on more responsibilities without more pay or recognition?" one nurse asked me.

"Aren't there other satisfactions to be had than money?" I shot back.

"Look, Tilda. Money's an issue. Deal with it. I'm getting thirty-three dollars per hour and I am not going to do more than I'm already doing in the ICU. I'm not going to read X-rays or write orders. I'm not going to examine the patient and explain to the first-year resident what needs to be done. If they want more from me, they'll have to pay me."

"What about professional development and job satisfaction, don't they count for anything?" I asked, but my question met with a torrent of protest from others who gathered around us.

"If they think my knowledge and skills are valuable, then they should pay me for it," one nurse said. "The doctors are getting paid more, why not us?"

"It's like during SARS. For three days I looked after a SARS patient and not one doctor came in the room to examine him. I told him how the patient was, I wrote the orders, and the doctor co-signed them."

"Don't nurses have enough work to do without taking on some of the doctor's role, too?"

"But other professions will take it on if we don't and you know what we'll be left with, don't you?" someone countered. "We'll lose even more nursing jobs. Other professions will take over."

"Is our hold on this profession so shaky that the only way to prove ourselves is to be like doctors?"

"If the public really knew what nurses did, they'd want our salaries to be commensurate with the stakes and the responsibilities we take on."

After listening to their concerns, I realized that finally, we had arrived at the frontier of the last taboo: it wasn't sex or death or poo – it was money. If we were *virtual* nurses – nurses virtually acting like doctors, yet not being formally recognized as such, nurses virtually being doctors' eyes and ears, rushing off here and there – *and* if we also were expected to be so *virtuous* – noble, angelic, altruistic, and sweet – how could we care about something as crass as money?

But here's my two cents for what it's worth: I believe we have come far enough that we can have it all.

15

NURSEZILLA

I have never felt I needed a break from the ICU, but when an opportunity came up to try something completely different, I was surprised at how fast I grabbed it. The job advertised at the back of a nursing journal sounded fun and easy, with lots of benefits: *Wanted: Registered nurse with fun-loving personality who wins trust, to work with children ages eight to sixteen at a summer sleepover camp in the beautiful Haliburton Highlands.* In exchange for providing basic first aid as needed to 350 campers and staff for four weeks, my own kids would get to go to camp for free. There would be a doctor from the local town on call and should a serious problem arise, there was a hospital forty-five minutes away.

"I love camp," said Terry White, the director of Camp Gitchee-Goomee at my job interview. His face could barely contain his broad smile and twinkling eyes. All of twenty-eight years old, he seemed like the quintessential "happy camper" himself. "I wish I could have gone to a camp like this when I was a kid, but my folks couldn't afford it. You'll never find me in my office. I'll always be out on the lake with the kids or on the basketball court."

His grin lessened briefly to level with me. "The truth is, the nurse's role is hard work and long hours, but it has its rewards, as you'll discover. Your own kids will have a blast."

All in all, it sounded like a great arrangement and though I knew Ivan would miss us, the bonus he would enjoy of being able to get in a few extra late-night poker games and afternoon rounds of golf while we were gone would more than compensate for our absence. As for meals and the house, he was a much better cook and housekeeper than me, so I didn't worry about that.

"Our campers are healthy kids from well-to-do homes who sometimes get a little freaked out when forced to be unplugged from their electronic worlds and to deal with nature. It's quite a shock to their systems," Terry continued. "Another thing I should mention is that we have a few campers with special needs. One boy is in a wheelchair and comes to camp with an attendant. There's a diabetic teenager who's on an insulin pump, and a child with mild autism."

"No problem. I'm sure I can handle anything that arises." I sounded and felt confident. "I know what an emergency is and what it isn't, and as for kids with special needs, as a parent, I know every child's needs are special, at least to that child and parent."

My answer seemed to please him. "Spoken like a true nurse and mother, too. In fact, your skills as a mother will come in as handy as your skills as a nurse. The camp nurse is a mother figure, *in loco parentis*. Sometimes all the kids need is a hug or a shoulder to cry on."

I understood that. It's exactly what I needed most of the time, myself.

"Homesickness," the director said, walking me to the door at the end of the interview, "is usually the main complaint. It seems to underlie almost everything the kids come to the infirmary for."

I knew a thing or two about homesickness. I'd had a bad case of it myself, all my life, especially when I had been at home. Problem was, I still didn't know how to treat it.

My kids were excited about going to camp. Max was a good swimmer but had never swum in a lake and he fretted about that. Harry bought a net on a long rod and was eager to start catching bugs and butterflies, or better yet, frogs. It would be a great adventure for them and I was pleased to be able to offer them this rich experience that I had missed out on. My parents never allowed me to venture out into nature. They considered the outdoors an uncultured, irrelevant place – not to mention dangerous and dirty, too. My summers were spent with safe books in clean hospitals and libraries. But I wasn't going to allow my own kids to be as deficient in this area as I was. They would learn to water-ski, sail, steer a canoe, pitch a tent, build a fire, and hike through the forest. Most of all, I hoped, they would learn to love nature.

A few days before camp started, I went to the camp office in the city to review the health forms that the parents had sent in ahead of time. There were no surprises in the medical section: lots of hay fever, some food allergies, a few kids with well-controlled asthma, and a girl who had to wear a patch for a lazy eye. They were healthy, but in the section where the parents were asked to list their concerns, there was quite a number and variety of responses:

Chloe refuses to eat fruit or veggies . . . Stacey is not to play any sports because she is clumsy and breaks bones easily . . . Ronald's father passed away and he has had bereavement counselling, but sometimes cries out in his sleep, otherwise okay. Gets a bad rash if he sits around in a wet bathing suit for too long and has an intense fear of raccoons . . . Please allow Jordan to use the infirmary bathroom for Number Two. If, after an hour, he still has difficulty, give him his Game Boy for as long as it takes . . . Raul stutters. Please place him with a patient, sensitive counsellor and discourage him from wearing girls' clothes . . . Stephanie has a fear of buttons, zippers, and snaps. No life jackets, please, or Velcro only . . . Sam needs to watch his vocal cords, please minimize his screaming and shrieking . . . Debra is afraid of thunderstorms, spiders, mice, and waterskiing and she gets some sort of reactions, but we don't know to what . . . Amanda usually loses weight at camp, must be weighed every five days, many food issues. Please remind her to say bedtime prayers and catechism on Sundays . . . Daniel has been seeing a psychologist for obsessive-compulsive disorder and has fears that relate to safety and danger. He must know that plans are in place for emergencies, for example, fire drills . . .

Yikes! These were *not* the so-called "special needs" kids. These were the "normal needs" kids! They weren't dealing with illness or disease, only with daily life and now, on top of that, being away from their homes and families. I was beginning to have an uneasy feeling. What had I gotten myself into? Give me septic shock, pulmonary edema, or fulminant hepatic failure any day. I could recognize a skin erythema, but had no idea what a poison ivy rash looked like – much less the plant that caused it in the first place.* Besides, I wasn't sure I was doing everything correctly with my own kids, much less someone else's. It was as if my practice in the ICU took place at the narrow end of the funnel of the health-care system. Now, I would be at the wide end, attending to the ordinary – as well as extraordinary – things that poured into the open mouth of the funnel.

A GROUP OF COUNSELLORS waved their arms in welcome as I reached the gate of the camp property. "The nurse is here! The nurse is here!" they called out. I had told them ahead of time what car I was driving. Their recognition of me was not due to any cartoon image they might have had of a camp nurse in khaki shorts, with a whistle on a string around her neck, a clipboard in hand. I wore a white peasant skirt and a sparkly T-shirt and had lots of luggage, including an electric fan, a radio, a deck chair, a fluffy purple rug, a case of Coke, and an ironing board.

A long, dusty road led to the centre of camp, where, high on a hill, was the main office and beside it, the infirmary cabin. At the back of it was my room with a view of the lake. I stood on the hilltop, breathing in the air that smelled and tasted so fresh. I could hear the wind rustling in the trees. I looked out over the whole camp, right down to the waterfront and the rippling lake. It was beautiful. Nestled in the trees were the campers' cabins, and one

---

* FYI: Red-tinged, three-pronged, droopy leaves.

for arts and crafts, one for "campcraft" (s'mores, campfires, tying knots, the camp brochure explained), another for ceramics. Rimming the edge of the campgrounds, from one end to the other, the lake sparkled in the sun and invited me to jump in – but not just yet.

Terry met me at the office and took me to lunch in the huge dining hall that had a stone fireplace and large bay windows overlooking the lake. It was noisy, teeming with kids chanting camp songs and cheers and acting out different parts of the songs. Conversation was impossible over the din but later the kids at my table introduced themselves and it turned out they were in fact counsellors, heads of water-skiing, "tripping" (hiking and canoe trips), and arts and crafts. I felt old. Compared to them, I *was* old.

After lunch, I unpacked. I was nervous and excited, but the calming breeze coming off the lake, whispering through the pine trees surrounding the cabin, was so relaxing that I fell onto my cot and into a deep, refreshing sleep.

THE NEXT MORNING it rained and the only visitors to the infirmary were the small group of campers I would get to know well over the next three weeks because I would be seeing them every day, three times a day, for their medication for Attention-Deficit Disorder, ADD. They received their pills on outstretched palms, swallowed them without water, and were quiet and polite, but the parents stated on their health forms that without those meds, they were hellions, out of control, hyperactive, fidgety, and unfocused. Yet Damian, Stephanie, Jackson, Dustin, and Greg were the sweetest, most docile kids I'd ever met. (Well, Greg seemed a bit wild, but I figured it would take him a little longer to settle into camp.)

Otherwise, there were no "patients" on that first wet, grey morning, so I busied myself by tidying up and scrubbing the floors and cupboards, which included removing a few mice skeletons left over from winter merry-making. I made up the four beds with crisp white sheets and organized the supply of common medications for aches, pains, coughs, colds, nausea, and allergic reactions. I prepared first aid kits to distribute around camp and for the trippers to take on canoe trips. I unpacked the dozens of emergency epinephrine pens – a veritable "epidemic" of epi pens – that had been sent to camp by worried parents. Though none of their children had ever actually had an anaphylactic reaction, the parents sent the pens, just in case. We'd certainly be well equipped in the event of an emergency. The infirmary was clean, organized, and well stocked with Band-Aids, sunblock, insect repellent, tensor bandages, sanitary pads, aloe gel, and a hot water bottle. I was ready.

BY THE SECOND DAY of camp, I recognized my regulars who came for their meds. I especially liked blond-haired Jackson. "Hey, d'ya wanna see my pet snake?" he greeted me.

Were little boys still getting mileage from that old chestnut? I decided to play along. "Yeah, sure, Jackson, I'd love to see your pet snake. Why don't you take it right out?" I folded my arms across my chest and waited. From the pocket of his jeans, he pulled out a live, bright green snake and I backed up.

"Don't worry. She's harmless." He cuddled it close to his face and the forked red tongue flicked in and out. "I find her every year. This is my third time. She waits for me. Her name is Rosie."

By the third morning, things picked up. A mild sore throat, two headaches, a bloody nose, and a tiny burn on a pinkie finger from an ember that had blown off the campfire the night before. I dug out a sliver from a finger and examined a camper with a history of asthma who sounded "tight."

"Where are your puffers?" I asked.

"In my friend's knapsack."

"Where's your friend?"

"On a hike."

I gave him another one to use until he got his own back and made a note to myself to follow up. I could see I was going to have to stay on top of some of them and be a bit of a nag.

By day four there was a steady steam of blisters, scrapes, cuts, bruises, and always a few kids with vague complaints of aches and pains. I gave them a hug or we sat and talked and they went back to their cabin. Some kids wanted Band-Aids, ointments, and painkillers, and other kids with similar sores, even ones encrusted with blood and dirt, cleaned them up with their own spit and kept on going. As far as I could tell, they all healed about the same. My own preference was to clean them, but I disliked Band-Aids. I hated coming upon them later that day or the next, floating in the lake or over the drain in the showers.

By the fifth day, there were more sore throats, headaches, stomach aches, and fatigue, and I began to see an emerging pattern, but was interrupted just then by someone shouting.

"Help! Where's the nurse?" It was Greg, one of the boys with ADD. "I can't feel my arm," he groaned, cradling his right arm in his left. "I'm paralyzed."

He sat down and I examined his arm. There was complete range of motion and it looked perfectly normal. Nothing seemed out of the ordinary with his arm, but he could use a shower at some point. "What happened?"

"I rubbed up against a tree," he said, crying out a little and jumping up and down. I cleaned the area and put a Band-Aid on it. "I might die," he moaned.

"You'll be fine," I said, patting his shoulder.

"It might get infected. People can even die from being tickled. You can die from laughing too much."

"No laughing for you for the rest of the day," I said in as stern a voice as I could muster.

Another problem was that the swim test jitters were going around camp. Not everyone took to the lake like a fish to water. They wanted swim excuse forms. "That nurse is mean," I heard one say after I refused her the note and told her to go change into her bathing suit.

So far, the camp's youngest kids, the seven- to nine-year-olds, rarely came to the infirmary. The teenagers required the most attention, along with a few counsellors. Sarah, the dance instructor, worried me. She came after every meal to weigh herself, and as far as I could see, ate only tuna and lettuce. She looked anxious. "I can't stop weighing myself," she admitted, "then I get angry at myself for whatever I've just eaten."

I looked at her robust young body, bouncy breasts spilling out at the top of her leotard, and her pretty, downcast face. I asked her about the cute guy I'd seen her entwined with around camp and she said it was Sean the head tripper and yes, they were a love connection. I'd caught sight of them late one evening behind the canoe shack, he clearly appreciating her curves, even if she couldn't.

"Do you want to talk about it?" Did she want me to make a referral to a counsellor or therapist in the city? Would she go see a doctor or a dietician to discuss her issues?

"I'm okay," she insisted. "I used to have an eating disorder when I was younger, but I'm good now." I guess I didn't look convinced. "No worries," she added with a forced smile.

By the end of that first week, I felt like a real camp nurse. All that was left was to call reveille at the crack of dawn, start barking out orders over the chirping of crickets, lead the sing-songs around the campfire, and take them on a ten-kilometre hike. I was actually enjoying myself.

At the end of each day, I fell easily into a deep sleep, but almost every night there was at least one knock on my door. Often it was Melanie, who had nightmares or anxiety attacks that made her feel like she couldn't breathe. Sometimes she just wanted to hold on to her epi pen, she said, as if it were a teddy bear. Sometimes a cup of hot chocolate or an overnight stay in the infirmary was all it took. Another night it was a counsellor who had gotten hit in the knee at a soccer game. I trudged out of bed and flip-flopped to the freezer in my pink Hello Kitty slippers. I was sleepy and my hair was a mess. "Please excuse my appearance," I said as I bent down to examine his knee.

"Don't worry," he said agreeably. "I have a mother at home. I'm used to what they look like."

I slapped a bag of ice on his knee and returned to bed.

"Feels great, Nurse Buffy, Camp Nurse Slayer," he called out to me after a few minutes and discharged himself, "I'm good to go."

But apparently not good enough because an hour later, he was back.

"Hey, Nurse Buffy, now I got hit in the balls with a ball."

"Ice!" I yelled out without getting out of bed. "Get it yourself."

"Sounds like a plan," I heard him mutter as he bashed into the refrigerator and helped himself to one of my Cokes.

EVERY MORNING, before the mosquitoes and the kids descended, I started the day with a long walk. I felt happy, useful, productive, and awake to this new world. One morning I looked up into a tree and saw a blue jay that I recognized from the Toronto baseball team logo. I walked past a farmhouse along the road just outside of camp and suddenly came upon a deer, strutting out in front of me, her baby close at her heels. *Bambi and her mother!* I would know a bear (Yogi Bear) but had no idea what to do if confronted with one. A moose I would recognize from the Canadian quarter coin. Spiders I spared because I considered them all descendants of the gentle, wise arachnoid whose ingenuity and generosity had saved Wilbur the Pig in *Charlotte's Web*.

ON THE FIRST DAY of the second week, there were still a few campers who balked at getting into the cool lake. I had to admire one boy who showed up daily, determined in his pursuit of a swim excuse note. On the third day his beguiling smile finally did me in and I wrote him one, warning it was the last time and that everyone had to learn to swim at some point.

"I knew you'd cave." He grinned and bounced out of there, prize in hand.

That day dragged on, interrupted only by macaroni and cheese and popsicles for dessert. After lunch, it rained again. The kids stayed in their cabins. I sat at my office desk and rifled through the huge drug compendium. I twisted a few paper clips. I thumbed through the local telephone book and noted with amusement that there was actually a Mr. Harry Potter residing in the nearby town and a Ms. Julia Roberts who owned and operated a beauty salon. I stretched out on the worn couch and listened to the raindrops on the roof. I heard a sound that I think was a chipmunk. There were major gaps in my outdoor education, but surely camp would rectify that situation. I was drifting off and didn't even try to stop it . . .

There was a knock at the door.

"Come on in," I called out and sat up on the couch. What time was it? Who knocked, anyway? Most of the kids just barged right in. An obese, freckled, red-cheeked boy of about thirteen stood there in long, baggy shorts and big shoes, the laces undone. "Hey, Nurse Tilda, I'm Mitchell." He stood on the porch at the screen door, looking worried.

"Come in and sit down." I sat up and moved over to a chair to let him sit on the couch.

"How are you doing, Nurse Tilda? Do you like camp? I hope you're enjoying camp," he said. "The nurse last year left after two days."

"Yes, I am. How about you, Mitchell? Are you enjoying camp?"

"Yeah, it's sweet." He looked to see if I bought that line. "It's really good. Well, good-ish."

"What do you like about camp?"

"The food." He brightened at that. "The tuck shop."

"Are there things you don't like?"

"Nothing really, except that I don't want to go on the canoe trip."

Aha! "Is there anything in particular that worries you about the canoe trip?"

He fell silent. "Not really." He sat slouched deep into the couch.

"Anything else bothering you?" He shook his head, but I sat quietly waiting and it came.

"Well, about a gazillion things."

"Such as?"

"I hate camp. My parents send me because my behaviour sucks at home, but I didn't want to come this year."

"This is your fourth year at this camp. Does this time feel different?"

"There's a big difference between being thirteen and being like fourteen, you know. When you're thirteen it's the beginning of being a teenager, so that's sweet, but like once you're fourteen, you're all grown-up."

"I see." Oh dear, the infirmary was starting to fill up now that the rain had cleared. I could hear them gathering on the porch.

"Mitchell, I'm pleased you've come to talk to me. You can come to me anytime with anything that's bothering you. The canoe trip is not for another week. Let's talk more about it later, okay?"

"Please don't call my parents. They're on vacation in Colorado, white-water rafting, and you'd have to speak to my grandmother. If you do, tell her I'm having a great time."

There was plenty more to talk about, but at that moment, Bill, the camp's handyman, burst through the door with a wound on his hand that was gushing blood. No Band-Aid for this one! I slapped clean gauze over it, showed his wife how to elevate it and put pressure on it, and the camp director drove him to the hospital for stitches and a tetanus shot. No sooner had I done all of that than thirteen-year-old Melanie rushed in, crying.

"I'm having an allergic reaction! I need my epi pen or Benadryl or something!" Her face was scrunched with fear and streaked with tears. I took her vital signs and her heart rate, blood pressure, and breathing were all normal. Her chest sounded clear. "What happened?" I asked, removing the blood pressure cuff.

"Someone was eating a nectarine and it sprayed on me. I'm having an allergic reaction."

She looked perfectly fine. I put my hand on her shoulder. I put her down on one of the beds to rest, close to where I could keep an eye on her. An hour later, she felt ready to rejoin her cabin.

After dinner I walked over to check in on Mitchell in his cabin. He was playing a card game with his cabin mates and when he saw me, flashed me a thumbs-up signal to indicate he was feeling better, but still, I planned to keep a close eye on him.

OCCASIONALLY, I TRIED to get a glimpse of my own kids, but Harry ran off when he saw me coming because he didn't want any preferential treatment. Max gave me a hug each morning at breakfast and I didn't see him again until the evening. They passed their swim tests with flying colours.

Despite my afternoon naps, I was tired at night and afraid I would sleep through a knock at my door. So I always left my radio on softly and kept the walkie-talkie with its occasional bursts of static, by my bed, just in case. I had no trouble dropping into a deep sleep each night, but just before I did, I took a moment to look out of my window. Fireflies darted by. I marvelled at a sky so full of stars. The lake was a glossy sheet, frosted with ripples, illuminated by the light of the moon. One night a bat swooped past me and I congratulated myself on not screaming. How brave I was becoming! I heard a bird and looked into the tree branches. It hooted again, and yes, it was an owl! Maybe one day I would reach the pinnacle of the great outdoor tradition: I would become a tripper – a strapping, hearty legend.

Midway into the second week, the after-breakfast line-up of miserable-looking kids was growing. The porch and waiting room of the infirmary were filled with campers, all dressed in baggy sweatpants, cozy hoodies, thick, grey woolly socks, and Birkenstocks or Crocs. They regaled me with their woes all at once and quickly figured out that the more tragic and urgent-sounding their malady, the higher up in triage they might rank.

"My mosquito bites are huge and they're keeping me up all night. I didn't sleep at all."

"I touched a poisonous frog and Jamie said I'm going to die unless I get the anti-venom."

"I've got a splinter and it hurts sooo much."

"My finger is infected." A girl pushed forward to show me. With a glance I could see it was not, so I put her at the end of the line. "Maybe it's broken?" she asked, to improve her standing.

What was provoking this onslaught of neediness? After determining there were no real emergencies, I treated the littlest ones for whom waiting was the hardest and then turned to Paul, a fourteen-year-old who had tripped over a rock and had a painful, slightly swollen ankle.

"Can I play soccer later?" he asked after I removed the ice pack.

"I'm afraid not. No sports for you today." I wrapped his ankle snugly with a pressure bandage and sized him for a pair of crutches.

He fell back against the couch. "What am I going to do all day?" he moaned.

"How about arts and crafts? A deck of cards?" *Dare I utter the dreaded word,* book?

He looked at me. "Your childhood must have been so boring." His eyes filled with pity. "No computers, no cell phones, no video games. What *did* you do all day?"

"Well, it was rough." I stifled a laugh. "There were hardships, but we had great music."

"That's true," he agreed, and strummed a few bars of "Smoke on the Water" using his tennis racket as an air guitar. They all seemed to be into classic rock 'n' roll – Led Zeppelin, The Who, and the Stones – and took great delight in discovering them.

Next, I saw a little boy who I had been following for a flare-up of eczema. I examined his arms, elbows, and knees. Ouch, I thought, looking at the red and painful-looking rash.

"Could you please try to be more positive?" he asked me ever so politely. "It helps me if you don't seem worried when you look at my rash."

Touché. Point well taken.

"Next!"

But how sick could they be, really? I wondered as I eavesdropped on snippets of their conversations taking place out in the waiting room.

"Who's brushing their teeth this week?" a counsellor asked his brood.

"When are you going on a day off, Jackie?" a little girl asked her counsellor.

"Tomorrow, sweetie, and I can hardly wait!"

"When do *I* get a day off?" her little camper asked, with such wistfulness in her voice.

"Doggie breath. Is it worse in terriers or poodles?" someone asked, but I didn't hear the answer.

"Jasmine, the swim instructor, is so hot!"

"Yeah, let's cover her with ketchup and get one of the trippers to lick it off!"

"Yeah, how 'bout we start a rumour about her and spread it all over camp!"

"Let's find two frogs and make them get married." Two girls were sitting on the floor, playing jacks. I hadn't ever seen that game played before.

"My mom's a forensic pathologist!" one girl told her friend.

"Mine's a chiropractor and a video maker," the other said. "Actually, I have two moms. The other one is a criminal defence lawyer."

"What are you into?" Two quiet kids from one of the older cabins struck up a conversation.

"I'm into cartooning."

"Oh, animé?"

"No, manga."

Perhaps the infirmary was the camp "water cooler," I thought as I taped and iced, bandaged, soothed, cleaned, hugged, examined, and listened.

OTHER THAN INCLEMENT WEATHER, the only thing that deterred campers from visiting the infirmary was the tuck shop. The two afternoons when tuck (candy) was given out I hid in the office and had time to myself. I hoped I was being sympathetic enough to their complaints, but my work with critically ill patients for so many years had hardened me to life's common problems. With my own kids, I have always tried to help them deal with life's discomforts, not avoid them. I want to spare them the pain I'd endured of being overly sensitive. Even as toddlers, if they fell I waited in the wings to see their reaction and went to them only if they called for me. If they needed me, I comforted them, but only then. The joke in my own family was not to bother Mom if a cut is merely bleeding or dripping. My kids know only *gushing* blood catches my attention.

The vast majority of kids at camp seemed to be having a wonderful time, but there were a few, just a handful really, who were miserable. Those were the ones whose worried faces I saw over and over again, and all my hugs and words of encouragement weren't making a bit of difference. Yet, when I brought them into my office, shut the door, sat them down, and gave them my complete attention, it was amazing what came out. They all got up afterward feeling, if not always "cured," at least better. The listening and paying attention were the treatments themselves. I figured that out when the girl with the "infected" finger came back the next day to show it to me again. "Now, is it infected?" she asked hopefully. I took a quick glance, again said no, and got instantly zapped by her angry face.

"Come here," I said more kindly. I took her finger in my hand and brought it, together with her, closer to me and into a light source. I examined her perfectly normal finger, then the other nine, then her hands and arms, and looked into her now-smiling face. *Ahh, I get it. She thinks I'm treating her finger, but I'm really attending to her soul.*

I became known as "The Splinter Queen." I developed a gentle, but sophisticated technique using a twenty-five-gauge needle to "de-roof" the skin over the splinter. If I took the time to examine the patient, scrubbed up like I was about to perform surgery, cleaned the site thoroughly, and distracted the kid with a few jokes, I had those mini-logs extricated in no time. A dab of Polysporin on the spot and I sent them on their way. The Splinter Ceremony became my specialty.

But there were some kids whom I couldn't "cure." They came almost every day to the infirmary with long faces, complaining of stomach aches and headaches, yet later the same day I would see them kicking a soccer ball or climbing a tree. If they caught sight of me walking past, their bright, smiling faces would suddenly droop. Jenny was one of them. Her throat was sore, or her head hurt, and she wanted to go home. I gave her the grape Tylenol until it was all gone, then the orange, then the bubble gum flavour. She confounded me because when I saw her around camp she was playing, dancing, even water-skiing. She had lots of friends, yet the moment she saw me she left them and came over. "I don't feel well," she said, her face instantly doleful.

On a visit to camp, the doctor told me it was called somatizing, displacing and sublimating. "They don't know how to express their feelings. It's easier for them to point to a physical discomfort rather than an emotional one. What they want from you is mothering, in the absence of their own mother or father."

I had no trouble giving that warm, fuzzy mothering touch to them. I felt for Mitchell and knew he was probably uncomfortable being overweight and unable to keep up with the others. Sarah, the dance instructor, had anxiety and possibly an eating disorder. I was even fond of Greg, the kid with ADD who, despite his daily meds, was still off the wall, loud, and disruptive, but quite endearing. He came in almost daily with minor complaints. When I read in his chart that his father had recently died, I asked him about it.

"Things happen," he said like an old, wise man. "Them's the breaks. But take a look at my toe. Is that gangrene? Do you think you'll have to amputate?"

My heart was soft to them all. They were all, myself included, city slicker kids dealing with communal living, bug bites, and food that wasn't always delicious and like what they ate at home. When they were cold, they didn't know how to warm themselves or how to get dry when they were wet. They didn't know how to calm or comfort themselves. They didn't have a place in their minds where they could go to work things out. They didn't know how to make themselves feel safe. I understood these things intimately. I had had to learn to calm myself, so that I could be calm for others. I had had to comfort others, even when I felt no comfort. Once again, I sat down to leaf though those health forms to try to understand it all.

> Jenny tends to be lazy, will complain of a stomach ache if she doesn't want to do something. Will go to the nurse even when there's nothing wrong. She is not to sleep beside Ellie. Have her bunk beside Michelle . . . Regarding Ryan's health: 1) He tends to get rashes. 2) His younger sister died two years ago. He has been dealing with anxiety related to this, and is unwilling to discuss it with anyone. . . . Catherine has weak sphincter tone. Her poos may come out without warning. I will send lots of extra underwear. Please make sure that she is not teased because of it . . . Cheyenne is physically inactive, tends to gain weight at camp. Please weigh her weekly and make sure she doesn't spend the whole summer reading comic books in the cabin . . . Trey is a sleepwalker, lower bunk please and

vegetarian, too. Has yet to establish close friends at school. Perhaps at camp? . . . Becky is big for her age, v. well-developed. Prefers to play with boys. She must practise her bat mitzvah portion twice per week, please check . . . Counsellors, please brush Lianne's hair every night (she has a lot of curls, but just hang in there, brushing has to be done). And teach her how to ride a bike . . . Darren has problems with speech articulation and needs to work on body awareness and space issues. Parents divorced, currently not speaking to his father. Occasionally gets migraines and will describe a fizzy, ginger-ale-type feeling in his head, or as if a bug is overtaking his brain.

Finally, by the end of the second week of camp I was able to match up names with neuroses and faces with fears. And as for the kids with "special needs," I hardly ever saw them. I waved at the kid in the wheelchair when I spotted her on the tennis court. The autistic kid was doing fine. I finally met the diabetic camper, but only because he came to the infirmary to refill his insulin pump. Those kids loved camp; it was the healthy kids who got sick or were unhappy. They were the ones trawling for drugs, pills, creams, or bandages for any and every deviation from their usual state of well-being.

Most afternoons, I stuck a note on the door: "Infirmary closed. Nurse on walkie-talkie for emergencies only," and snuck away. I went for a swim or a walk in the woods. I needed time to sit and think, to read, and take care of myself. Once I swam out to the raft in the middle of the lake and stayed there, treading water. Soon, a crowd gathered on the shore, signalling madly for me to come back. "What's wrong?" I called out to them.

"Shannon threw up."

They could probably deal with it themselves, but I turned back and headed for shore. It was often difficult to find a quiet moment to myself. Even though there wasn't a scheduled after-lunch clinic, if I was in the infirmary, sure enough, they would come. I'd be sitting doing paperwork and would hear the porch door open and close and soon they would turn the radio on to a rock station. The air

conditioning and my stash of popsicles and Gatorade was irresistible
to them. One afternoon, on a beautiful sunny day, the infirmary was
filling up. They waited for me, playing rock, paper, scissors, telling
jokes, and reading out loud the juicy bits from the sex ed booklets
I'd put out for them. *That's it, I've had enough.* I got up and switched
the radio to the CBC.

"Eww . . . what is that freakin' music?" someone said.

"It sucks big time," another voice agreed.

Thank you, Rimsky-Korsakoff, I thought as they fled, screen
door banging behind them.

BY THE END of that second week of camp, we were well into a swel-
tering heat wave. At breakfast I got up to the podium and launched
into a lecture about sunblock, hats, and water bottles. They booed.
Yeah, right, they grumbled. *Get real.*

The next morning I chose an adorable volunteer, the littlest
camper from the youngest group, the Purple Cabin, and spoke into
the microphone. "Lucy will demonstrate what to do in this hot
weather." She bounced up to the front of the dining hall. She put
on her baseball cap. She unhooked her water bottle from her belt
loop and took a long slurp. Everyone clapped. The Turquoise,
Maroon, and Silver cabins hooted and whistled. "Woo-hoo! Way
to go, Lucy! You rock, girl."

I returned to the microphone and waited for the noise to settle
down. "If you want to feel well and stay healthy in this heat, let's
see those hats and water bottles. Thank you, Lucy."

They clapped and then pressed in a throng all trying to leave
the dining room at once.

"That nurse is mean," I heard someone say.

"Yeah, she's pretty tough."

By noon, they started staggering in with flushed faces, headaches,
and heat rash.

"Where's your hat, your water bottle?" I asked Greg, who
usually talked a mile a minute. He looked pale and lethargic.

"I wasn't thirsty." He stretched full out, taking up the entire couch. His lips were dry and cracked. "I don't like the taste of camp water. At home, I only drink bottled water."

"It doesn't matter. You have to drink, especially in this heat."

"I'm not thirsty. I don't feel good." He lay there, unmoving. "Water is so not fun to drink."

"Here," I handed him a glass of red Gatorade, "drink this."

"I think I'll pass."

"C'mon, Greg. You need fluids in your system."

"I don't feel like it."

"Then you leave me no choice." I picked up a needle, grabbed his arm, and pulled it toward me. I snapped on a rubber tourniquet above the elbow. The other kids looked on, horrified.

"Hey, what are you doing?" He pulled back, but I hung on tight.

"I'm looking for a vein to start an intravenous. No one's getting dehydrated on my watch!"

"I'll drink!" he said, chugging down the Gatorade plus a glass of water before bolting out of there.

Well, I said to myself, that just proves that you can lead a horse to water, and you *can* make him drink! Yes, I was getting a bad rep. They had even given me a scary nickname: Nursezilla. It came about when I gave a child two tablets for a headache and next thing I heard was "crunch, crunch," followed by a long wail. I'd forgotten to tell her they weren't chewables and the bitterness made her retch.

Jasmine, the pretty swim instructor, was there and laughed. "We'll have to call you Nursezilla, the nurse from hell." I must have looked upset because she hastily added, "Just joking. It wasn't meant as a diss."

Yes, I had to control and patrol them, mother and monitor them, nurse and nag them. I was friend, police officer, mommy, rule-maker, and enforcer. I was constantly picking up pieces of expensive clothing left behind at the swim docks, the infirmary, or the dining hall. I would find articles of Gap, Roots, and Banana Republic clothing, most of them with name tags carefully sewn onto them by someone's parent or, possibly, maid. "Who belongs to this gorgeous Lululemon yoga shirt?" I said in the dining hall, holding up the wrinkled, soiled garment that someone's parents paid eighty dollars for. "If no one claims it, I'll enjoy wearing it." They groaned and laughed me off.

I knew I didn't stand a chance of being cool in their eyes, but I disliked the idea of being the nurse from hell. I came up with a plan. I took a drive into the nearby town. At the Giant Tiger – "Your All Canadian Family Discount Store" – I stocked up. Red licorice and Smarties and a bulk-sized bag of Skittles. The green ones would be for homesickness, one to start with, two if it was a severe case. Red ones for headaches and upset stomachs. Yellow for cuts and scrapes, purple for mosquito bites, and orange for whatever ails ya. A bag of lemon-and-honey-flavoured hard candies for the kids with sore throats. I went to the dollar store and bought some decks of cards, a bunch of *Archie* comics, a plastic game of checkers, and a metallic dart game to keep them busy in the waiting room. *I'll show them who's the mean nurse.* On the way back to camp, I stopped to pick up a few counsellors who were hitchhiking back to camp from town.

"What did you guys do on your day off?" I asked.

"Sleep, just sleep," they said, and to see their refreshed faces, I believed them. Playing is not as easy as it looks. Sleep was a precious commodity at camp and sometimes the infirmary was a hotel where they could crash and catch up on rest. (The time when the Copper cabin of older campers was caught streaking and were sent to the infirmary overnight was meant to be a punishment, to separate them from their cabin mates, but it turned out to be a cure. By morning, they were the most well-rested kids in camp.) Camp went at a frenetic pace and there was little downtime.

THE CANOE TRIPS were planned for week three. Most kids loved them, but some did everything possible to get out of going. I had been counselling Mitchell and he agreed to give it a try.

"Camp is about conquering your fears. Learning new things," Terry said firmly, backing me up. "It's the reason we don't let the homesick ones go home, unless the parents insist."

They were gone only three days, but when the buses started rolling into camp, bringing them back from Algonquin Park, I eagerly rushed down to greet them. I missed them. I was particularly anxious to see how Mitchell and a few others had managed.

"I swallowed a live minnow!" hollered Greg, the first one off, leaping from the top step of the bus.

"Technically speaking, that means he's not a vegetarian any more!" shouted his buddy.

"We got to see two frogs getting married!" said the girl who had been looking for that very thing, but her friend corrected her, "I think they were only engaged."

They clambered off the bus, messy, dirty, sweaty, smelling of bonfire and looking spotty with mosquito bites and splotchy in areas missed with sunblock, but they were healthy and happy. Standing around in groups, boys and girls together, they were laughing and telling their stories. Even those who had been nervous and reluctant returned to camp triumphant and pleased with themselves.

The last one off the bus was Mitchell. He came down one step at a time, dragging his knapsack behind him. At the bottom, he stopped and leaned against the bus. I went right over to him. "Mitch, how was it?"

"Awesome," he said uneasily, "but I feel bad."

"Come with me to the infirmary."

His counsellor took me aside. "No offence, Nursezilla, but he stunk up the whole bus. We could barely breathe."

I went to get a thermometer and when I returned I knew what the problem was. "Mitchell, do you have diarrhea?"

"No," he said. "But my stomach hurts. Could I sleep here tonight?"

"Yes, if you need to."

As I made a bed for Mitchell in a separate room in case what he had was infectious, I went back to him. His stomach was rumbling loudly. "Mitch, there's the bathroom."

"Thanks, I'm good."

"Are you sure you don't have diarrhea?"

"No, I don't." He looked so embarrassed. I cringed for him.

"Okay, Mitchell. I'll leave you alone."

When I came back later, he seemed to have fallen asleep but his stomach was still gurgling.

"Nurse Tilda?" he said softly.

"Yes, Mitchell. I thought you were sleeping."

"You know what? I have diarrhea."

"I thought so, sweetie." I washed my hands, put on disposable gloves, gave him some Gatorade, turned his room into a gastro-isolation ward, and prayed I wouldn't get it too.

"Should I take medicine?"

"Not necessary. You'll probably feel better in the morning."

If he did, I'd tell him the joke a camper had told me the other day.

"Have you seen the movie called *Constipation*?" he'd asked.

"No," I'd answered, rolling my eyes at yet another scatological joke.

"That's because it's *not out yet*! How 'bout *Diarrhea*, have you seen that one?"

"Can't say I have."

"Oh, it's all over town!"

I stayed close by Mitchell for the next few hours, not because I was worried, but because I was fond of him. In the morning, he felt much better, and waved to me at breakfast.

That day at lunch there was an announcement of a swim marathon for the older campers, counsellors, and staff. It would be one trip around the entire lake: three and a half kilometres. I wanted to do it. I went over to the sign-up sheet on the bulletin board and put my name down. I wasn't fast, but I was strong and I felt fairly confident I could do it. I wanted two things only: to finish and not be last.

My son Harry and his counsellor were my spotters, following beside me in a canoe. "Go, Mom, go," Harry said in his soft voice while the counsellor crooned in a beautiful, bluesy voice, "Boulevard of Broken Dreams," by Green Day, and "You're Beautiful," by James Blunt, and then in deference to my venerable age, every single verse of "American Pie." I found those mellow songs surprisingly motivating for that slow, but steady swim. "You're doing great," he called out from time to time.

"You're going to make it." I listened to them and tried to find the coach inside of me. An hour and a half later, at the finish line, when I finally hauled myself out of the water, there were still a few swimmers in the water behind me. My legs were wobbly, but I'd made it and I wasn't last. We were all finding ways to triumph at camp.

I WAS HEADING INTO the home stretch. It was the first day of my fourth and last week of camp and as usual, the evening clinic was packed. There were kids coming at me from all directions, asking questions, and presenting me with their various aching body parts. That night there were the usual sore throats, blisters, splinters, ear-aches, itchy bug bites, two kids worried they had lice, and one with an ingrown toenail. Then I heard a soft moan and something in that sound that made me come running. Terry was carrying a little girl in his arms. It was Lucy, my sun safety poster child! "My leg hurts," she said, holding on to her thigh.

"What happened?" I asked as Terry laid her gently on the bed.

"I fell off the swing," she said calmly, "in the playground."

"Did anyone see you fall?" I looked around.

"I was there." Her counsellor squirmed and looked away, knowing she should have been supervising her kids more closely. "But I didn't actually see it," she admitted.

I examined Lucy's leg. The skin was intact. There was no wound or bleeding, no bruising or swelling, and no difference in size between the two legs. The pulses in both legs were strong and easy to palpate and she had no difficulty wiggling her toes. I made baseline measurements to follow any changes. Only when I asked her to move her leg did she wince in pain. Her blood pressure was normal and her pulse slow and steady. Otherwise, she looked com-fortable and refused pain medication. In the waiting room, the other kids clamoured and were getting impatient and demanding. Darren called out that he was getting the fizzy ginger-ale feeling in his head. Leslie, a counsellor, dropped by for her anti-depressant medication, and wanted to ask me a few questions, if I had a moment, but unfortunately I didn't just then, could she come back later? A little boy from the Silver cabin had a sore ankle, but I only had time to call out to his counsellor, "RICE! Rest and Ice," and toss him a tensor bandage, adding, "Compression and Elevation!"

I returned to Lucy. She was sitting up in bed, eating a bowl of Cheerios. Her leg looked completely normal, but she still couldn't move it without wincing. I was worried. I thought of the long, dark, bumpy road to the hospital for something that might get better on its own. Could it wait until the morning? I was still far from clearing out the infirmary and I had to return the calls of dozens of parents who had been leaving messages. Some of them I dreaded calling. So many were upset or dissatisfied or suspicious. One angry father wanted to know why no one was looking after his kid's rash he read about in a letter home. I had to return a call to Clare's mother, who was not happy with the message I had left on her answering machine, in which I said that Clare was enjoying camp. "Well, she'd better be enjoying it with what it's costing me, and her father doesn't pay a cent," was the mother's return message. Then there was the father of a camper who was a surgeon I've known for years at the hospital where I work. When I told him that Zoë had come in with another headache yesterday, but was fine today, he told me to arrange for her to come home to Toronto for a CT scan of her head. He left a message that if I didn't call him back by this evening, he would drive up there right away to examine his daughter himself. I figured these were the "helicopter parents" I had read about in a magazine at the dentist's office. They were over-involved, controlling parents who micro-managed their children's lives to ensure everything would go perfectly. They were constantly trying to pave the way for their children, keeping them safe or rescuing them. Very good, but how devastating if a child's expectation was for everything to go perfectly and mosquito bites happen?

I cleared out the infirmary as soon as possible. An hour later, when I returned to Lucy, she was sleeping comfortably. I examined her leg again. I felt all around and she moaned softly when I touched it in one place, about mid-thigh. Otherwise, it looked perfectly normal.

"Are you sure you didn't see anything?" I asked her counsellor, who was lounging in the bean bag chair beside the bed. "Did you hear a sound, like a snap or a crack?"

"No. I mean, I was right *there* and everything." She sat up and gathered her long, loose hair into a ponytail. "But I was, like, over at the slide with other kids, so I didn't see *exactly* what happened to Lucy, but like, all of a sudden she goes, *owww*, and I knew something was wrong."

I felt uneasy. It was after midnight. The drive to the hospital was winding, dark, and treacherous at night and it might be for nothing at all. I phoned the doctor on call.

"She fell off a playground swing?" the doctor asked. "And her leg still hurts after four hours with no physical findings?"

I agreed it didn't make sense. Was I missing something? The doctor said it was probably nothing and could wait until morning. "If you say the leg looks normal, just observe her overnight." He paused to reconsider his certainty. "The femur is the largest, strongest bone in the body. A fracture would be very rare. There would have to be major trauma. She would be in a lot of pain if it was broken. You'd see clinical findings." I heard him tap his finger against his lips. "Keep her in the infirmary and I'll examine her in the morning."

Who could sleep? I stayed by her side all night, popping up frequently to check on her. In the morning, bright and early, a few friends from her cabin came to visit. "How ya doing, Wonder Woman?" one asked. "You were like Tarzan!"

Tarzan? I listened in closer.

"I bet you're never going to do that again, are ya?"

I pulled out Lucy's health form. Her parents hadn't written any comments, but Lucy herself had. There, scribbled in her own handwriting under the section "Restrictions on Activities," it read: "I am I am I am. I am Superman. I can do anything." I went back to her. "Lucy, describe to me again what happened."

"She was on the tire swing," her friend piped up. "She was swinging and swinging, around and around, and then smashed into the wooden post."

Forceful trauma can shatter a femur! I splinted her leg and ran for my car keys.

At the hospital, a ward clerk who had just stepped away from her computer was walking past when something caught her eye on the X-ray viewing box. She readjusted her glasses and made the diagnosis. "That's a helluva broken leg!" The bone had cracked in two, leaving a gaping space in between. If one of those sharp, jagged edges of bone had pierced an artery, Lucy could have bled to death in minutes!

I rode in a two-engine prop plane from a nearby air strip, right onto the landing pad of Sick Children's Hospital and delivered Lucy into both the parents' and the orthopedic surgeon's arms. After surgery, she was fine and would likely heal nicely, but I would take longer to recover.

I was newly sobered with the weight of my responsibility. Clearly, children did not always fit textbook descriptions. A camp nurse had to be a detective, too, along with everything else.

THE LAST WEEK OF CAMP was quiet, as if the kids knew to back off, the nurse couldn't take any more stress. I strolled around camp and everywhere I looked, I saw kids laughing, smiling, and being silly. I relaxed and began to cajole them about some of the more decidedly *underwhelming* complaints:

"I can't stop coughing. Do I have SARS?"

"The pain comes and goes and moves all around my body."

"I got bit by the hugest mosquito. Do you think I might get West Nile?"

"A fly flew in my ear. It's buzzing inside my brain and making everything go kablooey!"

Greg burst into the infirmary. "I need a condom. Right away. You got any?"

"Why don't you come into my office for a talk?" I was able to call his bluff because I'd caught a glimpse of the two guys who had sent him on this mission, snickering behind the bushes.

"No, forget it," he replied hastily. He turned, ready to leave without his bounty, and then bolted.

But I'd finally solved the mystery of his ineffective ADD meds. His counsellor told me he'd caught him throwing them in the garbage can outside the infirmary. Somewhere in the forest there was a very well-behaved raccoon.

ON THE LAST NIGHT of camp, just before falling asleep, I listened to CBC Radio playing Poulenc's Concerto for Piano and Oboe. "A gorgeous, witty, and mysterious piece of music," Shelley Soames, the announcer, said. "Just like someone you'd like to get to know." *I was once like that, but now I am old and weary.* I wanted to get home. I longed to be with Ivan. I slept through the night uninterrupted.

The next morning, there were lots of tears and hugs as the buses came to pick up the kids for the drive back to the city. The mosquitoes, the blackflies, the wet towels, the monotonous food, and the homesick days were all forgotten now.

"I love you," two girls sobbed into one another and pledged, "best friends forever."

"Camp made me who I am today," said Sam, all of sixteen years old, as he was getting on the bus. It had been his last year as a camper. "Next year I'll be a counsellor."

"What was the best thing about camp?" I asked a few of them.

"I learned to ride a bike," Lianne said, her beautiful hair hopelessly tangled. "My mom will be so happy."

"Doing nothing," another said. "It's the best. And no math tutors."

"Making music," a young camper said, her guitar slung over her shoulder, "it's way better than downloading."

Sean, the head tripper, and his girlfriend, the curvaceous Sarah, who seemed to have reconciled, however temporarily, with her body's need to eat three meals a day, both came over to give me big hugs. "You're awesome, Nursezilla," Sean said.

Mitchell came over to say goodbye and give me a big hug. "You're the nicest person at camp, Nurse Tilda. By far the coolest."

My kids and I piled into the car with all our luggage and lots of woven, plastic key chains, popsicle-stick napkin-holders, and lopsided clay pots. The counsellors swarmed our car, shouting goodbye and blowing us kisses.

Terry said, "I know you worked your butt off, but I hope you had some good times, too."

"Of course," I murmured, starting the ignition. My car's gas tank was full, but I was running on empty; my personal reservoir was down to zero.

"Oh, one more thing," he said as he bent down to the car window. "Don't be surprised if you feel out of sorts for a few days when you get home. It's common to take a while to readjust to your real life in the city, after camp."

"I'll be fine," I said. "Thanks, Terry." I shifted into drive. I wanted to be home already.

"What about next year?" he called out. "You interested? The job is yours!"

"Call me in January!" I shouted back.

16

OFF-DUTY

Just as Terry predicted, I did have an unsettled, deflated sort of feeling for a few days once home from camp. I think we were all out of sorts, returning to the hustle and bustle of the city, its humidity and smog, and now having to cool off in chlorinated public pools instead of the pristine lake at camp. I was eager to get back to the ICU, catch up with friends there, and return to the familiar rigour of my work. Then, I got news that jolted me out of my malaise.

It was from Daphne Marcus, my old writing partner. We hadn't seen each other nearly as often as during those six continuous years when we met every week to write together. I still saw her from time to time at some of the poetry readings she gave around town and we always waved at each other at our gym, where she worked out regularly and I, sporadically. While I'd been at camp, she'd left a phone message to call when I got a chance, nothing urgent she'd added, but when I finally got back to her it was just in time because she was going into the hospital the very next day.

"I've been having difficulty doing my workout," she explained on the phone. "I haven't been feeling myself." It was strange to hear her complain of anything, especially something about her body. She had yearnings, quandaries, and quests, but never ordinary aches and pains. She said she had been having stomach pains and bloating and on the phone, I could hear she was short of breath. At the end of our conversation, she mentioned, almost in passing, that the doctor had told her she had ovarian cancer. She said it as if it were neither good nor bad news.

"Oh, how terrible!" I gasped. *Not the disease that whispers, the "Silent Killer," whose symptoms are usually only felt when it is too late to do much!* It was a terrible diagnosis, especially with such advanced symptoms. I was stunned.

"I'm having surgery tomorrow to remove the tumour," Daphne said calmly.

Did she need anything? I asked. Did she want me to take her to the hospital? Or be there with her after the surgery? No, Ken, her husband, would go with her, but she thanked me graciously. She just wanted me to know. She had friends all around the world, as well as lovers, muses, and fans, but she had not told any of them. I understood that with me she felt safe, not only because it was me, but because I was a nurse. I knew that she wanted me to be her nurse.

The day after her surgery, Daphne started on a course of aggressive chemotherapy. Two days later she was discharged from the hospital, and we met for lunch at a dingy, old-fashioned diner around the corner from her house. It wasn't our usual type of place, but she wanted to go somewhere she could walk to. She said she was going to walk herself well.

She looked as elegant as ever, in a tailored pantsuit and Gucci print silk blouse. Daphne was not beautiful, but had an arresting elegance, a naive sophistication that caught people's attention.

"All of this," she ran her manicured fingers through her lustrous, wavy hair, "is going to go." She gave a laugh, neither rueful nor grim, more amused, than anything. "I've already chosen a wig." She ordered weak tea because she wasn't hungry, and I ordered a pastrami sandwich, because, well, I was. She looked at me unblinking while I ate. I think my presence gave her comfort, but she may also have been composing a poem.

"How's your family taking this?" I knew them well. In her

poems she had described Ken as her devoted husband and her son, Daniel, just finishing high school, as brilliant.

"Daniel is angry." She pushed the tea aside and dabbed at her lips. She reapplied her deep, red lipstick, the signal that she was ready to soar into her world of words. She took out her notebook and a fountain pen, one with purple ink, and looked at me as if to say, *Where's yours?*

"Who is he angry at?" (I liked to write, too, but not nearly as much as she did.)

"At me."

"He's angry at you for getting sick?" I asked even though I understood all too well the range of emotions, from rage to love, which a child could feel toward a sick mother. I slathered more hot mustard on my sandwich, trying to obliterate the familiar, disturbing thoughts.

"He has a lot of reasons to be angry at me, but I must remain the mother."

"How do you manage that?"

"I let him say what he has to say and listen but don't always take it in."

She must have sensed my need for further explanation, despite her eagerness to start writing.

"If someone says something to you, you have a choice whether to receive it or not. If you don't accept it, it will never get to its destination."

She was often full of new-age wisdom that I usually discounted, but this actually made sense. "What did he say?" She never minded when I pried.

"He said, 'If you were to die tomorrow, I wouldn't feel a thing.' He said I had shamed him and had been disrespectful to his father." She picked up her pen. "I made a conscious choice not to take in his anger. I kept my cool."

Had she always been so wise or had illness turned her into a Buddha overnight?

"I let him get it all out and I listened. Daniel and I are very close, you know. Then he lay his head down on the kitchen table and wept while I read poetry to him."

"What did you read?" That, I had to know.

"Leonard Cohen."

Of course, or else John Keats, "Beauty is truth and truth is beauty."

"Especially now, more than ever, I am committed to optimism. I refuse to entertain any dire thoughts. My father always used to say, 'accentuate the positive.'"

If Daphne was afraid of what lay ahead, she was doing a fantastic job of hiding it. I couldn't imagine having cancer and being so serene. She seemed pleased with the way things were going and didn't appear to wish things were otherwise.

"The doctors told me my body is already responding to the chemo. They say I'm doing great." She opened her notebook.

As always, for Daphne, eating and talking were only preliminaries to writing. I doubted that even now there would be any disruption to her routine. I was certain she would continue her daily free-flowing "morning pages," her walks and weekly artist's dates with herself, according to the instructions in her bible, *The Artist's Way*, a book by Julia Cameron. In all the years we had written together, Daphne had never cancelled a writing session and had considered my occasional excuses flimsy. A migraine, the flu, even giving birth – bring the baby along! – none were legitimate reasons not to show up at the writing table. "If you want to be a writer, don't let anything stand in your way," she would say. She herself accepted the sacrifices necessary to create art and if forbidden love affairs, travels to exotic locales, long-distance relationships, or intense communion with other artists served her muse, so be it. She did whatever was required to nurture her artistic soul. Her duty was to herself as an artist.

My duty was to myself as a nurse – at least during "office" hours. When I was on, I was on, and when I was off, I made a point of being off. Outside of the hospital, I was a mother, a secret writer, and a big-time daydreamer. I didn't always welcome opportunities to be a nurse, off-duty. But as I grow older, there is less and less of a separation between my professional self and my personal self. More and more, being a nurse is part of everything I do, both at work and away from it.

But there were times when I wanted a break from the caregiver role. Once I almost ran away from being a nurse. I was standing in line at a grocery store and recognized the cashier as the wife of a man who died in the ICU. I wanted to abandon my shopping cart, turn and run, before she noticed me, but it was too late. She had been smiling broadly at other customers but when she saw me, her smile vanished. Buxom and short with blunt-cut blond hair, she had big, blue eyes that instantly filled with tears. "It's been years, and still I cry."

"Seeing me brings it back," I said. It was all coming back to me, too.

She nodded and kept up her work, scanning my eggs, cat food, and orange juice, but I could tell she was back with her husband in the ICU, when I was his nurse. "I think about him every day."

"Of course you do, Genya." How did I even remember her name after so many years? I also remembered her husband's name. It was Vladimir and he had been in his early forties, perfectly healthy and strong, before becoming terribly sick and weak almost overnight. He and Genya had a daughter, Tanya, who at the time was a teenager in a pink sweater, jeans, and running shoes.

"Will my Dad be okay?" Tanya had asked me the night he was admitted to the ICU.

I hadn't worked there long, but already I knew to choose my words carefully, both the ones I said and the ones I didn't. I knew that my words, tone, facial expression, and gestures would be observed and analyzed. I took a deep breath. "Your father is very sick. We are doing everything we can for him. The next twenty-four hours will be crucial."

My yogurt and carrots sailed along on the conveyor belt. "I live for my Tanya," Genya sobbed.

I remembered even more. Vladimir made it through that night and the next. Genya and Tanya stayed by his bedside, speaking softly to one another in Russian. Later, they fell asleep, their heads resting on either side of him in bed. I was also there the day he died and they threw themselves on top of his body, wailing and shrieking, trying to pull him back to life, calling his name, begging him not to leave them. For years I've tried to put it out of my mind –

there had been so many patients in between – but when Genya saw me, it all came back for both of us. I wanted to offer consoling advice, but the only thing I came up with was what Ivan always says, and though it sounds trite, it is the truest thing. "Life goes on, doesn't it?" Life did have a maddening habit of going on even after your world is shaken. You have to make a conscious choice to go forward – or not.

"You were a good nurse. I remember."

I thanked her but silently vowed not to return to that grocery store for some time.

Yet, on another occasion, I was thrilled to be recognized as a nurse. I was walking through a crowded shopping mall, eating an ice cream cone, when I heard someone calling, "Yoo-hoo, Nurse!" A woman rushed up and plunged right into me, grabbing my arm. "You were my nurse when I was in the ICU! It was you." I thought about denying the allegation since I had absolutely no recollection of her, even after she told me her name. "I'll never forget you," she said. "You were there when I woke up after my surgery. I was so embarrassed to, you know, and you helped me with the bedpan." She got really choked up. "I'll never forget it." Both my ice cream and I melted.

THAT SAME FALL when Daphne fell ill, there were many people around me who needed a nurse. A neighbour called to tell me she'd found a lump in her breast. I rushed a close friend's mother to the emergency department after she collapsed at home. A girlfriend was having anxiety attacks or perhaps indigestion, or gall bladder or heart problems – the doctors didn't know for sure. Another neighbour, an elderly man, had a stroke and I visited him in the hospital and fed him soup. Jenna lost her baby in the sixth month and ended up having a hysterectomy, putting an end to any hope of bearing a child. We all visited her at home while she was still on long-term disability leave.

By that winter, Daphne lost her hair, eyelashes, and lots of weight from her already ballerina-slim body, but she was finding new ways to be glamorous. She was excited to have been chosen to model for a poster at the local community centre of members using and enjoying the facilities. She felt certain her hair would be grown in by the time of the photo shoot that spring. The day I visited her at home, she was getting ready to go to a party despite her nausea.

"I'm hoping the dry heaves will ease up by tonight," she said.

"You have the energy to go to a party after a week of chemo?" I asked in amazement.

"I've always been taught that it is wrong to closet yourself away."

Daphne was doing well. She didn't need much from me, but I had a feeling the time would come when she would, and I tried to prepare myself.

"DO YOU EVER GET called on by friends and family – even strangers – when they hear you're a nurse?" I asked the others at work and then regaled them with a funny story about what happened to me on a flight with Ivan and the kids to visit family in South Africa. "Is there a doctor on board the plane?" the captain announced somewhere over Namibia. A few minutes later, he called out again, this time for anyone with a medical background or any knowledge of first aid. I got up and made my way down to First Class. There, I found a drunken man in an orange and black dashiki, hopping around on one foot, yowling in pain from a toothpick that was sticking into the sole of his foot. I yanked it out, splashed on some alcohol (the rubbing, not the drinking kind), bandaged it up, told him to see a doctor when he got home, and that was that.

Roberta didn't say anything, but I knew she had taken care of her father when he was ill and how she worked tirelessly with her two children who had severe developmental problems. However, she did tell us what happened on a recent vacation in the Maritimes. "We were on the Catamaran in Prince Edward Island and a woman heard me mention I was a nurse so she came over and asked me to change her dressing on an incision from a recent surgery. So, I went into the washroom with her and did it," she said with a shrug. "It was nothing."

I understood. Nurses are familiar strangers.

Noreen told me about her sister-in-law who lived alone and spent her days drinking beer and smoking cigarettes, barely moving off the couch. Noreen brought her a meal and when she was there noticed a strange growth on her face and that her belly was hugely swollen. She took her to the doctor who drained twelve litres of fluid from her abdomen and removed what turned out to be a benign tumour.

"Twelve litres!" I looked at the garbage can next to the sink. Twelve litres would almost fill it to the brim. It was an incredible story, but I had seen bizarre cases like that.

"It's obvious she can't take care of herself any more." Noreen pulled a face. "But I told Bill, your sister has got to move in with us. She can't live on her own."

Patricia is a nurse who has the caring gene in a big way, but she's not relying on heredity alone to pass on the tradition to her own children. She teaches them lessons in caring even though her oldest is not even eight years old. "I always say to my kids," she told me. "If you hear someone crying, stop and find out why. Find out how you can help. Life is not about the almighty dollar, buying another car or a bigger house. You are in this world to help others."

EXACTLY ONE YEAR LATER, Daphne's cancer came back. This time she had to return to the hospital and have a colostomy. All those years of working out, standing in her spot in the aerobics studio in front of the huge mirror, she had always taken pride in her flat, toned abdomen, where now there would be a hole and a bag hanging down. A Clinical Nurse Specialist came to teach her how to attach the bag and empty it, how to feel clean, and how to manage swimming, bathing, and having sex. "You'd be surprised at how many people are walking around with hidden scars, blemishes, holes, tubes, and appliances. People you may even know," she said with a smile that put Daphne at ease.

Two weeks later, I visited her again. "Daphne," I said when I saw her, trying to hide the shock I felt at seeing her swollen face, bloated belly, and grey complexion. I had seen *patients* like this but never a friend. "You . . . you look . . . you look . . ." *Terrible, was the truth*. I am a bad liar, inept and unconvincing. "You look . . . different from last time." Fortunately, at that precise awkward moment, I recalled advice that Renata, a nurse who had worked in this cancer hospital, once told me: *Rejoice in the smallest details. There's always something positive to say.*

Daphne was wearing a luxurious, cream-coloured terrycloth robe edged in black silk and lace. I complimented her on it and added, "It's good to see you sitting up in bed." Her face brightened. *Praise any achievement, however small.*

"And," I said, looking her over, "I see you're wearing your watch."

She said she was feeling nauseous and asked me to give her her medication. She must have forgotten that I wasn't on-duty, nor was I her nurse. I handed her the call bell and told her to call her nurse, but she was reluctant to do so. She said she didn't want to bother them. I knew she felt more comfortable with me and probably felt she had to be economical in her quota of requests. Most patients feel that there is a limit to what they can request of their nurse. We probably make them feel this way because there *is* a limit to what we can give, but there is no limit to what they need. It's understandable, but what I couldn't understand was my reluctance to become Daphne's nurse. I wanted only to spend time with her and concentrate on memorizing her because I was starting to fear that I might one day be in the position of only having memories of her.

After the nurse came and gave her an injection, I sat with Daphne until it took effect. At the same moment, we both heard the sounds coming from inside her robe. Her bag was gurgling. It needed emptying and she looked to me. She didn't want to call the nurse back. I understand, I said, and emptied her bag quickly and efficiently. I had never smelled anything from Daphne other than possibly a whiff of French perfume – and now, this.

Then she told me that her nurses were too busy to take her to the atrium courtyard to get some fresh air, and she desperately needed her daily walk. Would I help her?

I do not want to be your nurse. I clenched my teeth and kept my eyes down as I got her slippers from under the bedside table and pulled back the covers. We looked at her feet. Her long, slender feet that had always been turned out in perfect ballet position as she stood in her spot in the aerobics studio were now pudgy, bloated balloons, swollen with fluid.

"A nurse told me they wouldn't ever return to normal," she said with dismay. "I'm trying not to take in her words."

"Well, she doesn't know you, does she? She doesn't know that you're not the average patient."

Daphne loved that response. She excelled at being special. Being called upon to be special brought out the best in her. But there was an unmistakable change in her that day, I realized as I helped her to the bathroom, pushing the IV pole alongside her. She had become a patient.

After our walk to the atrium, we turned around and headed back to her room. The minute we got there, I couldn't wait to escape. I got up to go and pretended not to see the many other things that needed taking care of by a nurse, things that every nurse would jump up to fix. I was off-duty. She said she felt like she was going to vomit. I said goodbye. On my way out I told a nurse that Daphne needed her and rushed past the nurses' station before she noticed from my uniform that I was a nurse myself.

"I JUST GOT HOME from the hospital," Daphne sang into the phone, a few weeks later. She was back to her daily workouts at the gym, back to teaching her English literature courses. She sent me an invitation to the launch of her second book of poetry that was written in and inspired by the Moonbeam Café – the coffee house where we wrote together many times. She had inscribed it, "To Tilda – My great, great friend on the writer's path."

Another year passed and the photo gallery of gym members was unveiled. One of them was a full-length, life-size picture of Daphne with her new hair grown in, thick and wavy, wearing a black leotard and purple tank top. She looked even more lithe and gamine, with her long neck and large, wide-set eyes. In the photo, she had struck an irrepressibly exuberant pose with her left, writing arm flung high into the air.

One cold, snowy March day last year, when every cell in my body was telling me to stay put, stretch out, and read a good book, for some reason, I grabbed my gym bag and went. It was mid-morning by the time I arrived, and Daphne had already completed her workout and was at her locker getting ready to shower. She used to enjoy being naked in the locker room but now she had a towel wrapped tightly around herself to keep her colostomy bag out of sight. I waved hello but didn't stop to talk. As I stood at my locker contemplating the merits of the Stairmaster versus a few laps around the running track, Daphne came over to me, bent down, and whispered, "I can't stop vomiting. Nothing is staying down. Do you think it could be something serious?"

I sank down to the bench. *Here it is.* It likely meant one very serious thing, but I asked, "How long has this been going on?" Stalling, keeping my face perfectly blank, I prayed to be wrong.

"Two days. Even a sip of water comes right up."

I wished it were something she had eaten. If only it was a pesky case of gastritis or upset stomach, but I doubted it. "Is anything draining from the bag, either solid or liquid?"

"No."

"Nothing? Not even gas?"

"No, not a thing."

For years, we had talked of poetry and prose, roses, wine, and lace. Never did I dream that one day we'd be talking about shit. "Daphne, it could be . . ." *an obstruction due to a tumour.* "Perhaps you should see your doctor."

"Do you think so, Tilda?"

"Shall I drive you?" I answered, changing back into my clothes. Daphne was a reluctant driver, even at the best of times. That afternoon the doctor sent her for a CT scan. It showed her abdomen was full of tumours. He told her he could not offer more surgery, only another dose of gruelling chemotherapy. He admitted her and a nurse came to start an IV.

"Please put it here." Daphne made a graceful arabesque with her right arm to proffer it to the nurse while keeping her left one close to her body, hidden under the covers. Of course. It was her writing hand. "I have a belief that my pages will see me through," she said to me. "No matter what happens, somehow I will find the strength to write myself through it." She continued to set daily goals: her morning pages, first thing, and then three laps around the nurses' station, and meditation for one hour.

"You always were so disciplined," I said, noting immediately her displeasure at my verb tense and nostalgic tone. "I mean, you *are* so disciplined."

"I try to keep the dire thoughts at bay," she said to me once again.

"How do you do that?" I asked her, needing her to explain the seemingly simple precepts once more.

"I take in the positive energy everyone sends my way and flood my body and my mind with it. I pray a lot. Tilda, would you pray with me?"

Okay, I said, and did my best. Of course praying helps, I thought. At least it helps while she's still alive, but why was I such a skeptic? Why didn't I hold out for miracles? "What did the doctor say?" I asked, bringing the prayer session to an end.

"He said ninety-nine per cent of patients die after a second relapse such as this."

I pulled my chair closer even though it was already touching her bed. "He's given you a very big assignment." We sat and thought about the work ahead of her. I wondered if she would still be the star pupil, the exceptional one, the valedictorian standing first in her cancer class?

"What do you think, Tilda? Do you think I can beat this thing? Do you think I'll make it?" She closed her eyes to take a deep breath, then opened them to receive my response.

I had never been asked a harder question. I couldn't look her in the eye because if I did she would see that I thought she was going to die. Still, that question hung in the air between us. I wanted to give the best, kindest response, but also the truest. I looked at her expectant face. How cruel it would be to say anything that might dash her hopes.

To Daphne, giving up was the worst possible choice, but wasn't there a peace to be found in surrender? I am committed to look at life as truthfully as I can, but I had to respect her way. As a nurse and as a friend I try to treat others as *they* wish to be treated, not how *I* would wish to be treated. It's like giving a present: you don't give what you would like to receive; you try to imagine what the other person would want. I had to find a way to tell the truth, but which truth and how to tell it? I delved deep into the well of all that I have learned as a nurse and said, finally, "If there is anyone who can beat this, Daphne, it would be you."

She leaned back against the couch, pleased to receive the gift I'd offered.

A FEW WEEKS LATER, the hospital sent her home and the doctors told her they had nothing more to offer her except palliative care, but she was angry at the very suggestion. I went to visit her and her husband, Ken, told me that the tumours were wrapped around her entire intestinal tract, cutting off the circulation. She was receiving nutrition at night through an intravenous line called TPN[*] that he managed quite capably. Their living room had been transformed into a mini hospital suite.

"I wrote only one line today," Daphne said when she saw me. "Nothing feels like a poem."

Ken asked about the drain in her abdomen. "Sometimes it flows well, but other times it seems blocked." He was an engineer and needed to visualize the internal structures in order to understand their function. I drew a diagram of the anatomy of the organs and how the tumours obstructed the outflow of fluid. By positioning Daphne on her side, gravity would ease the pressure. We talked about the laws of motion and the impedance of flow, until he said he understood. I sat down on the bed beside Daphne, feeling proud of my small but useful contribution.

She rocked herself back and forth. Suddenly, she lurched forward for the plastic basin into which she vomited in an almost graceful way. Ken rubbed her shoulders as she heaved into the basin and then hurried off to empty it and rinse it out. I wondered if he felt any of that resentment that used to sweep over me when I had been home

---

[*] TPN is Total Parenteral Nutrition.

alone taking care of my mother, but he seemed wholehearted in his new role as his wife's caregiver. He had a few more questions and for those, he took me aside.

"They won't admit Daphne to the palliative care unit, because she wants to have the night time nutrition. I see their point of view," he said. "Why feed someone who is only going to . . ."

"Hospitals can't tolerate too much ambiguity or contradiction," I explained. "They can't work at cross-purposes. If Daphne wants to be fed, she doesn't by their definition qualify for palliative care."

"To her, palliative care means it's the end."

"Yes, and it also means comfort."

"What should I do if I can't manage with her at home?"

"Has she expressed a wish to die at home?"

He shook his head. "She doesn't believe she is going to die."

"Bring her to the hospital when she is ready or when you are."

I went back to sit beside Daphne.

"It's hard, Tilda," she said, shuddering as she reached for the plastic kidney basin. "My poems are from my old self and I am still giving voice to my new being."

I was leaving the next day for a family vacation and I wanted to say goodbye to her, but she wouldn't have accepted it. I believed it would be the last time I'd see her, but when I got up to leave, she smiled and said she'd see me soon. I saw that she was not afraid of dying because she did not think it possible. It was her ingenious way of keeping fear at bay. But it was only a few days later, during that vacation, that a mutual friend called to tell me that Daphne had been admitted to the hospital and had died there, that morning.

It's the Jewish custom to rush to burial in the belief that mourning cannot properly begin until the person is in the ground. I was too far away to attend the funeral, but I wanted to know the end.

"I went to see her yesterday," the friend said. "I asked her how she felt. She said 'grand,' and then a minute later she died. That was Daphne, elegant to the end."

EVERYONE HAS SOMEONE they are worried about. Everyone needs a nurse, or will at some time. And once you become a nurse, or choose to act like one, you've signed on for life. Can you ever be off-duty? Once you know what you know and once you have chosen to care, can you ever look away and not respond when needed? Is it possible to turn off that awareness of others' needs, especially if you have the skills or knowledge to mitigate another person's suffering? It is, but you don't. For most nurses, their profession defines who they are. They are nurses everywhere, all the time. There's no turning back. *Nurse* is noun, verb, and adjective. It's a job, but it's also a way of being in the world, on-duty and off, at work and away.

17

DANGEROUS ASSIGNMENTS

My day was not getting off to a good start. Usually, I leave myself enough time so that I can sit for a few minutes before work in the underground mall opposite the hospital. I like to take the time to pause and locate my calm centre that I vow to maintain in the face of the possible things in the day ahead that might threaten to disrupt it. That morning, I guess I hit the alarm clock snooze button a few too many times, and had to scramble to get dressed and then rush off to work.

Outside the front doors of the hospital, there was the daily gathering of die-hard smokers clutching their iv poles (urine bags dangling off the bottom) with one hand, their lit cigarettes in the other. (It's the only place they can go because smoking is banned inside.) As I was about to get onto the elevator, two men, their fat bellies pushing out under their flapping hospital gowns elbowed their way forward, cigarette packs in hand, eager to get outside for their smoke. "I'm on thinners," one was saying to the other. "How 'bout you?"

"Me too," his partner said. "Man, they do a number on your heart."

Riding up in the elevator, I was subjected to more snippets of dreary conversations.

"Our health-care system is falling apart . . . gone to rack and ruin."

"Forecast calls for rain," a voice said.

"What a dull morning," someone else said. "Not a bit of sunshine."

Maybe it's time to look for a new job. Why do I still work in this depressing place?

It takes effort to be positive. It doesn't come naturally to me. At times, it requires courage and imagination, neither of which I could muster during a recent period of disenchantment with my hospital world. I wasn't burnt out as much as tuned out. Coasting along, floating mindlessly, going through the motions, I gave safe and satisfactory care, but my thoughts were elsewhere, my heart empty; the zing was gone. I worked to pay my bills, no more, no less. Then a patient startled me awake. He was a nameless, homeless man in his forties who came in with a terrible diagnosis. It's the condition that causes the greatest suffering, requires the most painful treatment, and has the bleakest prognosis. To me, it's the worst possible diagnosis because it's the one I once had. I knew this man's problem so personally that I never believed a time would come when someone like me could offer anything to a person like him, much less the other way around.

"YOU LOOK TIRED, Tilda. Coming off nights?" someone asked in the locker room as I changed into my scrubs.

"I'm coming on now." I glared back at her. "Day shift." *Do I look that bad?*

"Ouch. Excuse me."

Since I was running late, I hustled off to the ICU, checked my assignment at the nurses' station, and headed straight to my patient's room. "How was your night, George?"

He leaned back in his swivel chair. "I worked all night to save this guy, even though I'm not sure we're doing him a favour. But he's finally coming around. Say, how are your muscles?" He playfully squeezed my biceps. "This dude's rambunctious. You may have to call a Code White for the security guards or else snow him with sedation." Then George dropped down to the more serious story of our patient. A street nurse found him collapsed in an alley, cold, emaciated, and hardly breathing. She brought him in her van to our hospital where he was intubated and ventilated. During the night, he kicked and punched everyone who came near him. He had pneumonia, but the medical notes stated the more dire diagnosis: Failure to Thrive.

The physical causes of failure to thrive, such as poor nutrition and dehydration, are easy to treat, but when failure to thrive is due to a loss of will or lack of hope, that's a case of pure despair, and what's the cure for that? I had a feeling that's what we were dealing with here. In the place of "Name" read "John Doe." "Home address" was blank. He was an alcoholic, IV drug abuser, and out on bail for assault. He had been attending a methadone clinic but had lapsed back onto heroin, cocaine, and crystal meth use – in short, whatever he could lay his hands on. Then he'd developed an untreated upper respiratory infection that in his debilitated state quickly led to pneumonia and brought him to us in the ICU.

I looked into the room. He was sitting up in bed, peering out to see who would be his nurse just as I was peering in to see who would be my patient. I didn't like what I saw. He was thrashing about and had a nasty look in his bleary eyes. His ribs stuck out as he leaned forward, tugging his hands against the restraints pinning him down. He whipped his head from side to side, as if trying to escape the tube that was sticking straight out of his mouth. He was trying to kick his legs, but they were held down tight. Despite the restraints, he was managing to create quite a commotion. George finished giving me report and stood up to leave.

"Good night," I said with a fake smile.

"Good luck," he said with a sympathetic one.

I paused to consider my options. No one would want to switch patients with me and it was far too late to secretly pencil in a different nurse's name beside this patient. If I had gotten to work earlier, I could have made the change and no one would have been the wiser. Another more energetic and motivated nurse could deal better with this patient than I. I've done my time with difficult patients and the younger ones need this experience, I reasoned. Since I could see on the monitor that his vital signs were stable, I didn't go to him immediately. I sat outside his room, perusing the chart, and wasting time before I had to go in. Carmel, a nurse I'd worked with occasionally, came by with a guilty look on her face. "Hey, Tilda." She touched my arm. "I have a confession." She took up the seat beside me. "I got here early and saw they'd put me with this patient and I made a switch. I put you here instead. Have you noticed how they usually give the dangerous assignments to the black nurses?"

No, I hadn't noticed, but other nurses have told me this. Perhaps it's true, but what makes one assignment more unpalatable or difficult, or even more hazardous, than another? Caring for this patient was frightening for me for reasons no one could possibly know. It was my secret. The dangers here weren't only that this man was filthy, infected, and violent. I felt confident I could capably protect myself from those risks. I was far more susceptible to catching a lethal dose of his despair. I swallowed hard. "Carmel, if you feel you're being discriminated against, why don't you say something to the nurse who made up the assignment?"

She nodded but she seemed content to complain. "Tilda, are you okay with this patient?"

"Yes. No problem," I said, not letting on what I really felt, which was a sinking sense of dread. I got up. It was time to go in. I donned a mask, gown, and gloves to add yet another barrier to all the others that already stood between us. As soon as I opened the door of his room, I reeled back from the stench. I couldn't do my head-to-toe assessment, or check his heart rhythm, or listen to his lungs: hygiene was top priority. It would have to come first, admittedly, more for me than him.

He'd managed to wriggle out of all of his sheets, leaving himself exposed. Standing at the door, I could see the long red dotted lines of scabies along his legs and arms. His inner arms had raw, oozing purple-blue track lines along his veins. Whatever I felt or thought didn't matter. I filled a metal basin with hot soapy water. I got two more and filled them as well. More than ever did I wish I had that portable shower I had been dreaming up for years.

I stood at the foot of his bed. "I'm Tilda, your nurse," I said dully. *Lucky me. Lucky you.*

It's usually hard to make out the words of intubated patients but there was no mistaking this message. "Fuck off!" he mouthed, his eyes filled with rage.

I told him I was going to give him a bath, and he neither consented nor refused so I pulled the curtains closed and got to work. He was tall, maybe six feet, but all skin and bones. As I worked on him, he continued to thrash around, his fists clenched, still straining at the tube. Gradually, the water calmed him down a bit, but he kept shaking his fists at me. I was tempted to sedate him, but that might delay extubation. I wondered if loosening the restraints would calm him down but I was afraid to get hurt. I have received punches and kicks from patients and I realize that it is delirium that makes them combative, but still, it's not easy. I looked down the hall for help, but everyone was busy. I had to take a chance. As I untied one hand, he grabbed my arm in a tight grip. I shook it off. "Let go of me," I shouted, jumping back. "Don't touch me!" I threw the washcloth into the basin, splashing water all over the bed. "Are you going to let me take care of you or not?" He nodded and I released his legs. He kicked them around, perhaps just to feel them again after being tied down. I began to wash his face and neck with the warm, soapy water, maybe a bit roughly at first to show him who was boss, and then more gently. I shaved around his beard and then soaped up his arms and legs and chest and splashed lots of hot water all over him. I washed and combed his hair. He lay there, indifferent to what I was doing. Then I attacked the streaks of dried shit and urine that stained his genitals and legs. I have cleaned excrement from patients who were unconscious or who for other reasons had lost control, but this man had relinquished his continence. It didn't matter to him. It was the shit of not giving a shit any more.

I have never read much of the New Testament, despite the many copies that have been pressed upon me over the years by sincere and well-meaning Christians. But I knew that Jesus had washed the disciples' feet and that was a very impressive act indeed, although they probably weren't as dirty as this patient's. I thought about that as I washed his stinking feet, as I parted each toe and scrubbed away and tried not to look too closely at what I was pretty sure were bugs in there. I changed his sheets and put a fresh hospital gown on him. I pulled opened the curtains and didn't say another word or give him a backwards glance. I peeled off my gown and gloves, washed my hands, and hurried out.

PREJUDICE IS A TERRIBLE THING, but in a nurse it is unconscionable and dangerous. We hold ourselves to a high moral standard. Every professional does, but few are challenged in the way that nurses are to confront what most repels us. I once asked Tracy if there were patients she had difficulty caring for and she admitted, "I can't stand the way men in some cultures treat their women." She told me about a female patient who had tribal slashes all over her face and who had been circumcised. "I realize it's their culture, but it's too alien to me. I couldn't get past it and definitely couldn't get close." And when Laura had judgments about patients who made suicide attempts, she never showed it, at least not to them or their families. Noreen certainly hadn't recoiled from the hostile, angry family of Jerome, the young man who died of liver failure. Funny how Carmel, the one who complained that others discriminated against her, once complained to me about a patient. She told me about a new immigrant to Canada from Pakistan who was not yet a citizen but nonetheless was put on the list to receive a lung transplant. "Don't you think a real Canadian should get one before her? Not only that, but our tax dollars are paying for her health care! Don't you think it's wrong?" No, I didn't, but I had my own prejudices to contend with. Mine were against people who gave in to despair, just like I had.

It was when I returned home from travelling to Israel. I was twenty-four. My father had died, my mother was dying, I was estranged from my brothers, our house was sold, and I felt so bereft of family and comfort and all alone in the world. Friends offered me places to stay, but in my condition it felt like too much of an imposition. I was just as angry, just as homeless as this man. I had resources and supports but I chose not to turn to them. Instead, I went underground and hid. This man was me. I was him. I had been that lost, that close to the edge.

IN MORNING ROUNDS the team gathered to discuss his case. The staff doctor peered in through the glass. "He looks familiar," she said. "I've seen him before."

How could that be? He looked like any of them. He could be any of many derelicts loitering on Carlton Street on Sunday morning after a Saturday night binge or even that greasy bum near the University of Toronto who I used to rush past whenever he begged for a bus ticket.

"Where?" I asked her. "In emerge? The nurses there said he's a 'frequent flyer.'" I had obtained his old charts from medical records where it stated his name was Zbigniew Zwiezynskow, but there was no home address and no family, next of kin, or friends listed. He was all alone.

"No, I've seen him on the street, panhandling. Maybe around Yonge and Bloor."

It impressed me that she saw him as an individual, not as an anonymous street person. I, however, was not so noble. On the other hand, she didn't have to get as close to him as I did. She wasn't in his face as I had to be, breathing his air, smelling his pollution, hearing his grunts and obscenities. I was close enough to sense his thoughts, read his life story, and feel a bit of his pain.

When it was my turn to speak, I raised the question of whether he still needed the breathing tube. Initially he had required maximum support, but today he was more awake. Although his blood gases showed poor oxygenation, and he had a lot of thick, infected secretions, if we did a lot of deep breathing exercises and chest physio, he might be able to improve on his own. I suggested we extubate him and see if he would "fly." If he didn't do well, he would have to be re-intubated, but if that happened, then he could be sedated and allowed to get the rest he needed.

The staff doctor agreed. "It's worth a try."

The respiratory therapist removed the tube and I sat my patient up in bed and helped him cough out his secretions. He looked around, bewildered. "I need a drink," he muttered.

"Not yet," I said. "Easy does it." I put my hand on his shoulder.

We placed an oxygen mask on his face, but he ripped it off and threw it down on the floor.

Carmel popped in to ask me if I wanted to go for coffee with her. She must have been feeling guilty about her switcheroo, but it was karma: I was meant to have this patient.

"No, maybe later," I told her and sat down to think. I hadn't thought much about my own similarly dismal period in years, but now, taking care of this man who had nothing – no home, no family or friends – brought it all back to me. Eventually, I had decided I didn't want to live that way any more and faced the daunting task of taking up my life in my arms. The first thing I had to do was find a place to put myself, a shelter of some sort. "Home" seemed like an impossibility. I took the first place I saw.

"Donna! Get the screwdriver!" the landlord of Regal Mansions hollered down the hall to his wife. "The hacksaw, too!" Clearly, there were some loose screws, but I had no idea what this man was planning with the hacksaw. He led me down a dark, narrow hallway that smelled of cigarette smoke, cooking, and the bodies of the many lives living in the rooms behind the doors. It was dimly lit with shaded lights and sand-filled spittoons at the elevator. We stopped at the bachelor apartment for rent on the second floor. It was at the back of a three-storey building overlooking a parking lot. It didn't have a kitchen, only a tiny refrigerator and a hotplate in the corner of the room. There was only one rule at Regal Mansions, the landlord informed me: no pianos.

Drugs and guns are welcome, I suppose. "That won't be a problem."

It was in a rundown building in a seedy neighbourhood. "Toronto's twenty-fifth homicide of the year happened right around the corner," he boasted. The apartment was dirty and the walls were crumbling and needed paint. "It ain't the Taj Mahal, but if you get bored, you can go across the street to the church and watch the weddings."

Joy didn't hesitate to offer her opinion. "Don't even consider this dump, Tilda. Come stay at my apartment until you get yourself sorted out. I have a futon."

"I kind of like this place. It's growing on me."

"Yeah, it grows on you all right. Like a fungus."

I called the landlord to say I'd take it. I hired a painter, a Russian man who promised to do "special job for young lady." I handed up a cup of coffee and a doughnut in a paper bag to the top of the ladder and stood back to gaze around at my new periwinkle blue walls. It was the colour of dusk and dreams; of in between, of day turning into night and night turning into day. It was a *becoming* colour, I thought, pleased with the paint and my pun.

"Let me ask you something." The painter rested the roller on the can of paint. "What's nice girl like you living in dump like this? You should live with parents until wedding. What boy want girl who lives in bachelor apartment? A *parscutzveh* we call this type."

"I hear you," I sang out. "Thanks for the advice."

At night, I heard babies crying, people screaming, cats yowling, a dog's toenails clicking on bare floors in the upstairs apartment. Vibrations of Bob Marley and the Wailers thrummed through the wall and floorboards along with the earthy whiff of dope, when I left the windows open. I lay down on the bare floor so I could feel the warm throb of Jamaica in my bones. The smell of hot, steamed fish and fragrant jasmine rice permeated the hallway each evening as I trudged down the hall after spending the day with my mother. A Vietnamese family lived across the hall. There were about twenty pairs of plastic sandals and slippers outside their apartment, beside the front door. Once, when the door was open, I saw the family squatting on the floor in a circle, their rice bowls cupped in one hand, chopsticks in the other. I left the window wide open and one night a squirrel scurried in. I tossed him a few kernels of popcorn, grateful for his undemanding companionship. We were all looking for places to call home.

I bought a little travel alarm clock with green hands and numbers that told the time in Tokyo, São Paulo, and London. I took my parents' stuff out of storage and donated my father's clothes to a home for alcoholic and homeless men. I imagined the bums at the Silver Dollar Tavern on Spadina Avenue sporting my father's lime green polyester shirts, black beret, and paisley cravats. There wasn't anything useful like furniture or kitchen utensils, but there was a foot-long sign with my father's credo, THINK, in bold letters and his Underwood typewriter with the keys that stuck. A bunch of dried up ballpoint pens from dry cleaning plants and a stack of library cards from every small town he'd passed through. There was his Ponderosa Steakhouse discount card and a catalogue from a medical supply store featuring raised toilet seats and bathtub bars.

Joy came for a visit. "How's your new place?" She stepped gingerly over the threshold. "I'm so glad you're back. I missed you. We have so much to talk about," she said like old times, like we were fourteen again. She handed me a plant in a pot as a housewarming gift. I didn't want something I would have to take care of and she read my thoughts.

"It's a cactus, you goof. Put it on the windowsill and give it a few drops of water every other month. You can handle it. Cocooning is what you have to do now."

I had no curtains so I cut up green garbage bags and before taping them over the windows I caught a glimpse of a pretty garden in someone's back yard. It seemed unimaginable that I would ever sit in a garden like that with civilized people. Even with my garbage bag curtains in place, the sunlight filtered through along the sides, like shafts of light slicing through an aquarium. I slept on a mattress on the floor and didn't bother with sheets or blankets, just pulled my jacket over myself like I did when I slept in the park. *Home*, I kept trying out the word before I fell asleep.

One morning, I got up and went to the refrigerator. It was empty from the top shelf to the bottom. It was entirely up to me to make this place a home. I was coming to the bitter realization that the mother/nurse I yearned for was going to have to be me. It was up to me to fix myself – or not. I was tired of always being homesick. I had been yearning for a home for so long, even when I was at home. I got to work. That day, I scrubbed and scoured that place until it shone. In the evening I went out to buy bubble bath. The options promised were "revitalizing," "rejuvenating," and "soothing," but since I had no idea which remedy I needed, I settled on "moisturizing." I realized that the time had also come to buy a few groceries.

I HELPED MY PATIENT out of bed, eased him down onto a comfortable chair, and went back out to my desk and computer. As I sat there, I returned to the question I've asked myself every day of my life as a nurse. Do I love my patient? Some would say love is a lot – too much – to ask; only skilled caring and basic respect are necessary. Many would claim that love is not a requirement for the job. Nonetheless, it's what I've come to expect of myself. Because, after all, what is prejudice if not a failing of the ability to love? And if I couldn't manage love, at least I wanted to offer *loving kindness*.

I went back into his room and pulled up a chair and sat down beside him.

"What's your name?" I asked. "I mean how do you pronounce it?"

"Whaddya need to know for?" His voice was hoarse from the tube.

"What should I call you?"

"Nothing."

"Who are you?"

"Nobody."

I waited.

"Okay. Call me Joe." He picked his nose.

"How are you feeling?" I waited. "Joe?"

"How the hell do you think?" His skinny legs were splayed open and he scratched at them.

"Your legs must be itchy," I said, and he grunted. "I'll get you some cream for those bites."

"I'm thirsty. I could use a drink."

"How about some juice?"

"Got a beer?"

I handed him a cup of orange juice. He took it, looked at it, and hesitated.

"What's wrong?"

He turned meek, unsure. "Do you have apple instead?"

I stopped in my tracks. He'd found my soft spot. I preferred apple, too. We weren't apples and oranges. We were both apples.

"God, I need a fucking drink in the afternoon. I mean a real one."

"I know how you feel." I craved something in the afternoon, too. For me it was coffee or chocolate, or both, but wasn't it the same thing as booze or drugs? Both were cravings to fill the same emptiness. We each had our own drugs of choice.

"I'd like a smoke, too."

"Can't help you there. I'm sorry."

Perhaps this was compassion. It wasn't being upset with someone else and it wasn't fixing people's problems. It wasn't feeling what they were feeling. It was simply bearing witness to another person's predicament. For years I hadn't known how to give and always either gave too much and felt overwhelmed, or else gave too little and felt inadequate. So often, I turned away in the face of things that shamed or disgusted me, things that scared or saddened or enraged me. To be the kind of nurse I wanted to be I had to get beyond these barriers. This way of compassion empowered me. It felt healthy and helpful. For years I had been a caretaker and now I was a caregiver. Caring was no longer a burden. It was my life's work, the work I was meant to do. My emotions no longer felt like a liability. I was able to do this work *because* I care as much as I do, not in spite of it.

Joe and I sat together. There were questions I wanted to ask, advice I thought of offering, maybe even a pep talk. Instead, I sat quietly, giving him the space to speak if he wanted to, hoping my presence was some comfort. I wanted to tell him I had once been just as lost, but had found my way back. Should I have told him? Probably not. There was no need to say or do anything.

My shift was almost over. I asked someone to cover for me and raced to the bank machine and withdrew five twenty-dollar bills. As I slipped them into his worn, empty wallet, I knew my small gesture was a token, more for me than him. I said goodbye and went out to hand him back over to George, who arrived back for night shift. He would likely be transferred to the floor the next morning and eventually discharged back onto the streets to a men's shelter or detox centre. Like so many of our patients, once they go out the door we lose contact. Maybe he will get a dog or find someone to love. Love can bring about miraculous cures. I know this from personal experience.

18

NURSING CONFIDENTIAL

"Is it true?" Laura asked. "I heard you left the ICU. Have you finally come to your senses?"

"No, I didn't leave. I merely took some time off," I said, a touch defensively.

"After all these years, it's getting to you, isn't it? Face it, Tilda, it's time to make a change. Even Tracy's had enough. She left."

It was true. After completing her degree in nursing, working full-time in the ICU, and being a full-time hockey mom, Tracy resigned from the ICU and took a position as a public health nurse. I've been encouraging her to go on and do a Master's or become a Nurse Practitioner,* but she looks at me like I'm crazy. She's got a student loan to pay off, a mortgage, and kids going off to university next year. Her career has taken a different course. She's teaching mothers how to breastfeed and care for their babies and told me she's enjoying the new challenges.

---

* A Nurse Practitioner is a nurse with an expanded scope of practice who is qualified to diagnose and treat illness.

Every few months Laura's Line gets together. If more time goes by, I pine for them. I need to see them, be near them, and hear the interplay of their voices. Recently, one Saturday evening, we were sitting outside on a restaurant patio sipping drinks. We meet on weekends now that all of them, except me, work weekdays, nine to five. I asked Tracy about her new job.

"It feels strange going into people's homes. It's their territory. The other day I asked a mother how her baby was doing and she told me he'd gained two pounds since my visit the week before. I took one look at the baby and I was horrified. He had a bony, triangular face. I picked him up. There was no way that baby had gained weight! What could I say to the mother that wouldn't freak her out or make her lose trust in me? I asked her if I could watch him feed. I wanted to see the baby latch onto her breast and how he sucked. How many poos, pees, I asked her? She said she'd just fed him and she was putting him to sleep. But I had a terrible feeling. Something was wrong. Your baby needs to be weighed, I told her. I made her promise she would get him weighed that day. She said she would, but I worried. I called her on my day off. She ended up taking the baby to emerge and he had to be hospitalized. He had lost nearly three pounds, and finally she saw how serious it was."

We sat taking that in. Only then did we realize what this meant. Tracy saved that baby's life.

"A new nurse wouldn't know that," said Frances finally. "It takes experience and intuition."

Or a good teacher to guide her, I thought, looking across the table at Frances.

I'd been teaching, too. Back in the ICU, I had taken Sandy under my wing. (Her real name is Sankofa, she told me.) She's from Eritrea and has big blue eyes, mocha skin, frizzy hair framing her face, and a huge, beautiful smile. She is new to Canada, but is an experienced nurse who has worked in many countries – it seems that highly skilled nurses are in demand all over the world. She was paired with me in the ICU for a day and we were caring for a liver transplant patient, four days post-op. The new liver was not yet working optimally and there were complications. The patient's husband stayed by her side all day and the children were in the waiting room. Sandy and I ran the entire day, giving her blood transfusions, platelets, plasma, and medications. Later, her blood pressure dropped and her blood-clotting factors were so depleted that she started vomiting blood. Still, there was reason to believe her liver would recover with the whopping doses of steroids we were giving her. In short, it was an ordinary day in the ICU.

It was even becoming ordinary for her husband. "I've finally realized that every day is a completely different day here. It's a strange state of mind you have to wrap your head around," he said, nodding, "hoping and praying she's going to get better and preparing myself for the worst."

Yes, that about sums it up, I thought, looking at him. Sandy and I were on opposite sides of the bed. We lifted the patient up to place the X-ray plate behind her back and found a large pool of blood seeping out underneath her. We cleaned her up as best we could and I glanced over at the husband. He seemed to be coping, but Sandy looked horrified. It clearly wasn't an ordinary day for her.

"I could never work here," she said later, on a coffee break. "It's a scary place."

"You're right," I agreed.

"How do you cope with this work?"

"There is so much you can do to help people."

"Have you worked in the ICU long?"

"Twenty years."

"Wow," she said, looking at me. "You don't look that old."

"I don't feel old, but I started in my twenties and now I'm in my forties. Believe me, it happens fast."

The prospect scared her. I've seen this same surprised look in the eyes of younger nurses when they consider the possibility that such a thing might happen to them, too.

"Your real name, Sankofa," I asked, "I mean your African name. What does it mean?"

She smiled shyly. "It is difficult to explain. It may sound strange to you, but it means one who reclaims the past in order to move forward."

THE OTHER DAY I was about to get onto the elevator and I almost bumped into a very energetic elderly woman from Volunteer Services who was getting off. She was pushing a rickety cart out in front of her and it was the exact same size and shape as the one I used to fill with books and take all over the hospital. Near the bottom, underneath the patina of the thick, cream-coloured coat of shiny paint, there was a scratch and I could see a chip of the old bright blue paint. It was the same cart I used to push all around the hospital, thirty years ago! Now, it was loaded with Italian, Korean, and Chinese newspapers. No one in hospitals these days is well enough to read novels. If they're there, it's because they are sick and if you happen to catch one reading a book, it's time to send them home!

SOMETIMES MORE THAN a few months slip by between get-togethers with my gang, but we keep tabs on one another by phone and e-mail. Everyone's well, taking good care of themselves, despite a few aches and pains that have started creeping in. Last year, Tracy's mother died suddenly and she worries about her father now, left on his own. Frances took care of her older sister, who was ill for many years until she died a few months ago. As usual, we talk about work, the good old days, and new topics such as varicose veins, menopause, and kids.

"What did we used to talk about?" I lamented.

"Boys!" we laughed.

Frances and Laura never married and seem perfectly happy on their own. Laura did date a few guys, but stopped because, as she said, "They're all either looking for a purse or a nurse!" Life is good for all of us, but back then we had some of the best times of our lives. To be sure, we saw the worst things, but also the best. We helped people return to their lives, mothers to their children, husbands to their wives. We delivered good news with jubilation or bad news with gentleness. We used morphine to relieve pain and later discovered how we could bring about comfort with our touch, our words, and our presence. We saw things so raw and real we could speak about them only to one another. We exchanged wisdom, some of it practical and basic, some of it instinctive and complicated, some of it modern and sophisticated, and some of it timeless and ancient.

Tracy and I used to laugh about a plan we had, to cause a scene at a dinner party in which we would reveal the truth about our work. Everyone would stop mid-chew. They'd put their forks down as I would cheerfully tell them about the litre of pus we drained out of one guy's chest cavity. They'd weep as I would tell them about the tiny smile the semi-comatose man gave when his wife bent down to tell him she loved him. Their jaws would drop after I would tell them about a young man, a ward clerk, who was hit by a car while running out at lunch to register for university courses. In the afternoon he was declared brain-dead and became an organ donor and by that evening, another man dropped down to his knees in gratitude to that unknown donor and to God. Of course we never went through with our devilish plan, but I realized that when you put some things into words, they gain a weight and a power that they hadn't had when left unspoken or unrecorded.

"I hope you never do that." Frances was aghast. "It would be too unsettling for people."

"Hey, Frances," Laura interjected, never at a loss for a jibe at her. "Did you hear they removed the word *gullible* from the dictionary?"

"Did they really?" Frances asked. "Now, why would they do that?"

"Because it means the same thing as the word *Frances*."

"You're mean." She stuck her tongue out at her. "All I'm saying is there are some things you shouldn't tell people. It's too shocking. It scares them. Besides, they'd never believe you."

"You *should* tell people," Justine insisted. "The public needs a dose of reality."

"It's good Tilda's out there telling people about nursing," said Tracy. "Many people don't know what nurses do. They still think it's bedpans and helping the doctors."

"Yes, it should be Tilda, after all, she's still embedded with the troops, down in the trenches."

"So, Tilda, what else have you been up to lately?" Justine wanted to know.

I told them that I'd started working on my Master's degree and about the travelling I'd been doing across the country, meeting with nurses and speaking with them about our work and our stories.

"I hope you're telling them about all the exciting developments," said Frances, "like Nurse Practitioners, and clinical nurse specialists. Nurses are now First Assistants in the operating room."

"What about film studio nurse?" Justine said. "They need nurses on movie sets. I did that once and gave a Tylenol to Denzel Washington. I would have liked to have given him a lot more! Once, I got to airlift a patient to Anchorage, Alaska. What a blast! Oh, and make sure you tell them about the army. The army needs nurses. There are lots of wounded soldiers these days."

"I met a nurse who runs a sexual assault clinic, collects forensic evidence, and counsels victims," Tracy said.

"Remember those old Cherry Ames books, Tilda?" Laura was a big second-hand bookstore browser and had recently bought me two, in mint condition: *Cherry Ames, Jungle Nurse* and *Cherry Ames, Army Nurse.* "Even Ol' Cherry Ames would be shocked at what nurses are doing now!"

"What *do* you tell the student nurses you meet on your travels?" Frances asked.

"I start off by asking them why they chose nursing."

"I tell you what I'd say," Laura interjected. "The only choices open to me were teacher, secretary, or nurse. So I ended up being all three."

"Well, these nursing students say they've heard you make a decent salary and that there are good dental and drug benefits and lots of opportunities for advancement. I ask them how many plan to work in patient care when they graduate and they all raise their hands. Then I ask, what about five years from now, how many of you plan to still be at the bedside? You know what?" I took a breath for the clincher, "None raise their hands. They all want to be managers or researchers. Patient care is a stepping stone, an apprenticeship at best."

"It's understandable. Nursing takes a lot out of you. Not everyone can stay in it," said Justine.

"A friend of mine asked if I would advise her daughter to go into nursing," Tracy said.

"No way!" Laura interrupted again. "I hope you told her to steer clear of that!"

"Why?" I snapped at her. "Has nursing been so bad for you?"

"Listen, Tilda, young people these days want to have a life and can you blame them?"

"So, I told my friend," Tracy said firmly, to try to diffuse the tension, "I don't know your daughter, but how about your son? We need him even more. That opened their eyes."

"Yeah, so do you still think sisterhood is powerful, Tilda?" Laura put to me.

"Yes, I do, but maybe we have too much of a good thing. We need men to balance the mix. Nursing would benefit from the way men think and take action. I'll tell you one thing though, new nurses these days have no difficulty with computers or any of the technology that we will struggle with."

"Tell me about it," said Frances with a huge sigh. "The other day I was having a problem with the monitor in the CT scanner room. I called the technician and he explained to me how to fix it, but I couldn't get it to work and was getting frazzled. The patient's IV was going interstitial* and I had to spend all my time with the friggin' machine and on the phone with this guy. I said to him, please come in and see for yourself what the problem is. 'Oh no, no, madam. I cannot do that,' he says. 'I am speaking to you from Bangladesh.'"

"What did I tell you?" I said. "That wouldn't faze new nurses these days. They are completely at ease with technology. They know how to find information on the hospital database or the Internet and they think way more globally than we ever did. They're a lot more confident, too. Way more than I ever was," I added as an afterthought.

"You were one of the worst cases I've ever seen," said Laura. "You spent your first few weeks in the ICU running to the bathroom."

---

* Outside the vein.

"There's something wrong with a nurse who isn't terrified at first," said Frances. "It's a good sign." She smiled at me. "It means the nurse is motivated and wants to be safe. It means she realizes the enormity of the responsibilities we're taking on."

I looked at Frances's kind face and around the table at each of them. Did they even know how much I had learned from them and how much they had given me, not just as colleagues, but as friends, especially during a difficult period of my life? How could I ever tell them all of that or thank them or tell them what I really felt which was that I loved them?

"But it can't be easy for them, Tilda. The hospital is still a shock to most people," Frances said.

That's true, I thought, remembering Sandy's horrified face on her first day in the ICU. For most young nurses today, the hospital is still the place where they are confronted for the first time in their lives with people who are frail or hysterical, confused and combative, or lying in bed unconscious. They are expected to take care of bodies that ooze and leak, and that sigh and cry. "I feel for these new nurses. They start off with the best of intentions, but unfortunately, things happen along the way that wear them down," I said. "Generally speaking, people who choose nursing want to help others. By and large they are good, moral people."

"Things are improving," Frances said. "Nursing has come a long way. Back home in the Maritimes, when I did my training, a nurse had to get up to give her seat to a doctor. Now, nurses are diagnosing and prescribing. I heard a nurse on the radio speaking about organ donation after cardio-pulmonary arrest. And look at the nurses in the ICU rapid response team!"

"Nothing's changed," Laura grumbled. "Hospitals are dinosaurs. They're dying institutions."

I agreed with both of them. We did still need new ways to care for people in hospitals and in their homes. "We're stuck in the old tired way of doing things. The new ways aren't yet in place."

"I wonder what hospitals of the future will look like," I mused. "Do you think they'll ever really be patient-centred as everyone says they should be?"

"They won't be patient-centred until they stop being so

doctor-centred," Laura said. "In fact, if they were nurse-centred, everything would improve because nursing is about patient care."

"Yeah, doctors should lobby for more nurses. What they want for their patients will only be achieved if they work with us," said Justine. "I'm afraid to admit it, Laura, but I agree with you."

"I'm actually very easy to get along with." Laura leaned back and sipped her drink. "Once you people learn to see it my way."

Typical Laura.

I WAS INVITED TO SPEAK to a class of first-year nursing students. I stood at the front of the room and looked around at the young, mostly interested, a few bored, faces. It was still a sea of women's, mostly white, faces, but I've heard the trend is changing. Their pens were poised, ready to take notes. I got up there and introduced myself. I told them, yes, I'm a nurse, working at the bedside, caring for patients for more than twenty years. Their jaws dropped. I heard a collective gasp in the room.

Twenty years goes by a lot faster than you'd imagine it would. I stood before them, the old, sage, withered crone nurse they imagined me to be. They were eager to ask questions of a real, live working nurse.

"What if you disagree with a doctor's orders? Do you still have to do it?"

"No!" I practically shouted. "If you disagree with something, speak up, but be able to express your rationale and work out your differences."

"What happens if you make a mistake? Will you get fired?"

"Do everything you can to prevent mistakes by asking lots of questions and double-checking yourself and with a colleague if there's anything you're unsure of. If you make a mistake, own up to it by disclosing it fully. Learn from it and make sure you don't do it again."

"What do you say if a patient asks if he is going to die?"

I told them that once I walked by a patient's room and I saw Nicky with her ear down low, next to her patient's mouth as he lay in bed. I moved in closer to listen in. "Am I dying?" I heard the patient ask. Nicky paused and said, so tenderly, "Yes, dear, you are." I could see the connection between them that Nicky knew that was the right thing to say to that person at that moment. For other patients it would not have been appropriate. The hardest thing about patients dying is that it makes us face our own discomforts on the subject. "Work on yourselves to develop the sensitivity and wisdom to know what to say and do in each very different situation," I advised.

"What is it like when a patient dies?"

"At first, it may frighten you. It may bring up disquieting feelings about your own loved ones. In time, you'll learn to deal with those feelings. A patient's death may be a sad or joyful event or it may be peaceful or conflicted, but as a nurse there is so much you can do to make dying comfortable and dignified for the person and the family." *One day you may even grow to appreciate how lucky you are to be with people during these precious moments.*

"What do you do if a patient doesn't like you? Has that ever happened to you?"

"Never!" I joked, thinking back almost twenty years to Mrs. Wilson, stage name: L'il Roxy, and how I did everything I could think of to win her over and never did. "It's hard when patients are angry or hostile, but you will learn in time that, usually, it has nothing whatsoever to do with you. They take out their emotions on the safest and closest person – you, the nurse. You will learn how to set clear limitations and boundaries so you don't get hurt."

"How do you keep up your ideals?"

"I don't know . . . but they are stronger than ever." They waited for me to come up with a more useful sound byte. I dug deeper inside. "Sometimes you may need to step back from nursing and reconnect with the reasons you chose it. If you are in it for the pay cheque or the job opportunities, those things won't sustain you in the long run."

"Why don't nurses get more respect?"

"The onus is on us. We get as much respect as we show toward ourselves and our profession. Only when we acknowledge what we know and can offer our patients, when we conduct ourselves as professionals and use our voices to advocate for patients and speak out against injustices, will we get the respect we deserve. Our voices will be heard, but only when we speak up."

"What is the secret to being a successful nurse?"

"Find ways to enjoy it and make sure you have fun. Help your colleagues and accept help from them! Take good care of yourselves so that you can take care of others." I knew what awaited them, how frightening the hospital world can be, for patients, to be sure, but also for nurses. I owed it to these young, well-educated nurses to tell the truth.

"What advice would you have given to those students?" I asked Laura's Line that evening.

Frances started. "Don't try to be perfect. You can't fix everything. Do the best you can."

"Never eat pizza on night shift." For once, Laura wasn't sarcastic. "You'll regret it afterward."

"Have some laughs," said Tracy, and we had one remembering a night shift years ago when the song "Gloria" came on the radio that sat on top of the refrigerator and how Tracy suddenly jumped up, began to sing and boogie around the nurses' station like it was a disco, and how the rest of that night flew by.

"All very amusing, but I hope you told them the most important thing is that nurses have to get political," said Justine. "That's the only way we are ever going to improve things for our patients." Way back when I was still trying to figure out the difference between a vein and an artery, Justine was attending rallies and negotiating labour relations to improve our working conditions. "Think of the numbers," she went on. "There's a quarter of a million nurses in Canada alone. If only we were organized and stood together, our power to make changes could be immense." Then she turned to me. "How about you, Tilda? Isn't it time you moved on to bigger and better things?"

I knew what I wanted. "I'm happy where I am."

"Well, I hope you're telling people they'd better be nice to us," Laura warned. "Soon there's going to be another disaster, maybe sister of SARS or avian flu or bioterrorism, and who do you think will be taking care of the victims?" She surprised me with her next comment. "You won't catch me going to work when the next pandemic rolls along. I'm running for Algonquin Park, to wait there until it's over."

"I don't believe you," I said. "During SARS, you led the way! You were the first one brave enough to go into the patients' rooms." I can still picture Laura, covered from head to toe in protective gear and how she managed to reassure her patients with her eyes over the top of her mask. She looked like she had just stepped out of a spaceship on Mars. I can still see the curve in her back as she leaned closer to bridge the space between them. Her body said *I'm here with you. I'm not going anywhere. I have all the time in the world for you.* Laura had also managed to reassure the rest of us who were terrified to go in. SARS was lethal. It killed many people, including doctors and nurses, but Laura insisted that with the right protection, we would be safe. We are nurses, we have to take this risk, she'd said. We know how to go in safely. Now, she claims she'll run away? I don't believe her.

"Yeah, I'm tired of being a hero," she insisted. "I didn't sign up for danger duty and I have a feeling that SARS was just a practice in disaster. A dress rehearsal before the big one."

What had changed in her or was she bluffing? If the time came, I believed she would be there, as she was before. Nursing is in her blood. She's got a bad case of it.

"We'll see" was all she'd concede.

"What about you, Justine?" I threw back at her.

I'd never seen Justine so wistful as she looked at that moment. "When the tsunami hit South East Asia, and the hurricane New Orleans, I was envious of the nurses who went there to treat shock victims, set up health centres, give vaccinations and medications. That's what nursing is about."

I don't think we've ever gotten together without mentioning Nell. We still couldn't forgive ourselves for not recognizing her cries for help. "When Nell went to the hospital," recalled Frances, who had tried the hardest to reach out to her, "she wouldn't let me come with her, even though she said on the phone she was coughing up black sputum. She did tend to exaggerate at times."

"Yeah, just a bit," we chuckled.

Frances continued. "She told me that when she got to the ER

and saw how busy it was, she jumped off the stretcher and got to work, starting IVs and giving out meds until she eventually collapsed, but not before starting her own IV and giving herself an antibiotic, of course. I wouldn't have put it past her. She was an incredible nurse. That was the last time I heard from her."

I reached into my bag and pulled out my surprise dessert. It was a rare, limited signature-edition bottle of ice wine. The waiter uncorked it and poured for us. That afternoon I had heard a wine connoisseur on the radio praising this superb harvest and its peach nectar silkiness. I knew it would be the perfect complement to our summer-sweet friendship. The expert also said something that made me think of nursing. He praised the winery and explained how they employed the latest technology in the service of preserving traditional values of winemaking. Nursing must do that, too, I thought.

Why had so much changed? Health care is expensive and stretched to the limit, new technologies are available but human needs are still the same. Perhaps in our infatuation with technology, we have strayed too far from ensuring that people's most fundamental requirements are met: food, clean water, hygiene, relief, comfort, education, solace, safeguarding, monitoring, rescuing, kindness, human touch, and beauty – all within the domain of nursing. Whether it's cardiac nursing or pediatrics, public health or camp nursing, it comes down to these things.

I no longer differentiate between the person I am and the nurse I've become. Nursing is my profession and my way of life. It is a deep and abiding concern for the human condition. We are all nurses – or have the capacity to be – and we are all patients – or have the potential to be. I owe nursing a lot. It saved my life many times. Through the discipline of taking care of patients, I learned how to take care of myself. By finding compassion for my own suffering, I developed more compassion for others. Nursing showed me how to be joyful despite my own sadness. It has given me an awareness of the world's suffering and the skills and knowledge to do something toward its alleviation. It has taught me how to love things I never thought I could love. Nursing is my way of celebrating life. I raised a glass of the sweet wine and offered a toast to my sisters: "*L'chaim* – to life!"

ACKNOWLEDGEMENTS

Thank you to everyone at McClelland & Stewart, especially Marilyn Biderman, Jenny Bradshaw, Elizabeth Kribs, and Krista Willis.

Thank you to my patients and their families for the privilege of being your nurse.

Thank you to the entire team of the Medical-Surgical Intensive Care Unit, Toronto General Hospital. I am especially grateful to Stephanie Bedford and Edna Lee who made many improvements to this book. Thanks to Alexandra Radkewycz of the University Health Network for her assistance.

Thank you to my gang, who should know who they are, but here goes: Judith Allan-Kyrinis, Ann Flett, Chi Chi (Cecilia) Fulton, Lisa Huntington, Mary Malone-Ryan, and Linda McCaughey.

I am grateful to these mentors who helped make me a nurse and who continue to lead the way for so many: Virginia Bates, Sherrill Collings, Ingrid Daley, Mary Ferguson-Paré, Maude Foss, Doris Grinspun, Mary-Lou King, Marlene Medaglia, Denise Morris, and Kelly Sundarsingh. I would like to acknowledge Suzanne Gordon's insightful writing about nursing that has deepened and clarified my thinking on these matters.

Thank you to: Barbara Turner-Vesselago – I can't imagine a better writing teacher; Catherine Gildiner, who told me what this book was about; Rabbi Arthur Bielfeld, who raised questions that I tried to answer in this book – and for much, much more. Thank you to friends who have nurtured me and thus, this book: Elise Dinstman; Tony, Daneen, Jonathan, Noel, and Luke Di Tosto; Joy and Bunny Friedman; Anna Gersman; Vanessa Herman-Landau; Rivi, Alan, Yonatan, Omri, and Yarden Horwitz; Avery Kalpin; Cathy, David, and Rachel Kreuter; Tessie Oredina; Bob, Norah, and Robyn Sheppard; Chick and Dick Weiner. Thank you to my wonderful Israeli *chevrai*; dear Leo Baeck friends, especially: Maggie Atkin, Eileen Goldberg, Lesley Kalpin, Marcie Kisliuk, Rhonda Schlanger, Ella Shapiro, Lori Sugar, Laurie Waldman, and Shirley Weiss-Greenspan; and treasured BJCC friends: Larissa Ber, Nadine Cowan, Pam Glass, Mara Koven, Annie Levitan, Andrea Pines, Rhea Wolfowich, and in memory, Malca Litovitz.

I thank my family: Harry, snake charmer and lover of all things reptilian, who I hope forgives me for not writing a book about someone famous (Nelson Mandela or Wayne Gretzky were who he had in mind); and Max, artist and athlete, who has taken great care not to body-check me too roughly into the boards so that I might live to write this book. Most of all, I thank Ivan Lewis for everything, but especially for showing me the way to – in the words of Gustave Flaubert – "be orderly and disciplined in daily life, like a good bourgeois, so that I might be wild and violent in my art."